The NHS in the UK: a pocket guide 2007/08

Peter Davies

The ninth edition of *The NHS in the UK: a pocket guide 2007/08*.

First, second, third, fourth, fifth, sixth, seventh, eighth and ninth editions published by:

The NHS Confederation
29 Bressenden Place
London SW1E 5DD
Tel 020 7074 3200
Fax 0870 487 1555

To order further copies of this Guide or other Confederation publications, contact our publications sales team on
0870 444 5841 or visit www.nhsconfed.org/publications

ISBN 1-85947-136-6
Printed in the UK.

Design by Grade Design Consultants, London
www.gradedesign.com

© NHS Confederation 2007. All rights reserved. No reproduction, copy or transmission of this publication may be made without written permission of the publishers.

No paragraph of this publication may be reproduced, copied or transmitted save with written permission or in accordance with the provisions of the Copyright, Designs and Patents Act 1988, or under terms of any licence, permitting limited copying issued by the Copyright Licensing Agency, 33 Alfred Place, London WC1E 7DP. Any person who does any unauthorised act in relation to this publication may be liable to criminal prosecution and civil claims for damages.

All diagrams and charts reproduced herein are the copyright of the sources listed.

POC00301

Contents

Foreword	6
Sponsor's foreword	7
Introduction: one system – four structures	8

Part 1: How the NHS works

1 The structure of the NHS in England — 11

Parliament	11
The Department of Health	13
Arm's-length bodies	16
Strategic health authorities	17
Primary care trusts	18
NHS trusts	23
Foundation trusts	24
Care trusts	25
Children's trusts	26
Managed clinical networks	26
New providers	27
The role of boards	32

2 Where care is delivered — 39

Primary care	39
Community health services	48
Intermediate care	50
Secondary care	52
Mental health	59
Involving patients and the public	64

3 NHS strategy: putting policy in context — 70

The planning framework	71
Priorities 2005–08	75

4 NHS quality: improving healthcare — 79
Organisations' responsibility for quality — 79
Healthcare professions' responsibility for quality — 90
Feedback from patients — 95
Complaints — 96

5 Financing the NHS — 101
Sources of funding — 101
Resource allocation — 104
Capital — 109
NHS spending — 111
Buying goods and services — 118

6 Staffing and human resources — 121
Workforce planning — 121
Training — 124
Productivity — 127
Pay — 128
The NHS as an employer — 131

7 Information technology in the NHS — 133
National Programme for IT — 133
The electronic NHS — 139

8 Public sector partnerships — 142
Local authorities — 143
Other partnerships — 149
Public health — 151

9 The NHS in Scotland — 162
The structure of NHSScotland — 162

Strategy and policy	170
Financing NHSScotland	173
Staffing and human resources	175
Information technology in NHSScotland	177

10 The NHS in Wales — 180

The structure of NHS Wales	180
Strategy and policy	187
Financing NHS Wales	190
Staffing and human resources	191
Information technology in NHS Wales	192

11 The NHS in Northern Ireland — 194

The structure of the NHS in Northern Ireland	194
Strategy and policy	199
Financing the HPSS in Northern Ireland	201
Staffing and human resources	203

Part 2: Gazetteer

The NHS: a brief history	204
An A–Z of the NHS	210
Acronym buster	222

Index	231
Acknowledgements	236
List of advertisers	236

Please contact us on 020 7074 3325 for more information about the versions of the *Pocket Guide* suitable for those with a visual impairment.

Foreword

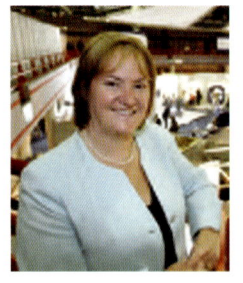

Welcome to the 2007/08 edition of the NHS Confederation's *The NHS in the UK: a pocket guide*.

In the 10th anniversary year of the NHS Confederation, the NHS is delivering more services, faster and better than ever before. The service has become complex, with many organisations fundamentally restructured and new technology changing the way we work. Whether you are new to the NHS, have years of experience or just need to know more about how the service works, this guide will be an indispensable aid to help you navigate through the system.

The 2007/08 edition of the pocket guide includes new sections on:
- the NHS' vital statistics
- commissioning
- reconfiguration latest
- Mental Health Bill
- NHS deficits (or achieving financial balance)
- efficiency and productivity targets
- progress on health inequalities.

Once again, the guide has been supported by advertising from selected organisations already working alongside the NHS Confederation and in particular Atos Healthcare, who have kindly agreed to support this year's guide. We are grateful to those organisations that are supporting the guide this year.

While over 90 per cent of patients rate their care as good, very good or excellent, the public perception of the service is significantly lower. This guide will give you the facts about how the NHS actually works. If you have any comments on the guide or suggestions for inclusion in next year's edition, please contact our publications team on 020 7074 3200 or email publications@nhsconfed.org

Dr Gill Morgan DBE, Chief Executive, NHS Confederation

Sponsor's foreword

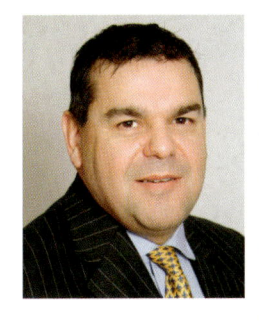

Atos Healthcare is pleased to support the publication of this year's pocket guide to the NHS.

The NHS and service providers like ourselves face real challenges in meeting public expectations of healthcare services and in creating the sustainable transformation needed to ensure their delivery. Reducing inequalities, improving performance and productivity, delivering innovative solutions that combine value for money with efficient services – these are the commitments Atos Healthcare shares with the NHS. However, these can only be achieved if all service providers work alongside one another to improve services to patients. Adopting a parochial approach in which providers work in isolation not only does a disservice to patients and taxpayers, it is also a disservice to other providers.

Atos Healthcare brings considerable experience in business consulting, IT solutions and medical services to the many parts of the NHS with whom we work at a local, regional and national level. Our aim is to deliver integrated healthcare services that support change, support staff and meet patients' needs.

We know from experience that those values are also shared by the NHS Confederation, and we look forward to the continuing transformation of healthcare services in the UK.

Mark Bounds, Senior Vice President, Atos Healthcare

Introduction

One system – four structures

The National Health Service is based on common principles throughout the four constituent parts of the United Kingdom, but its structure in each is quite distinctive – and increasingly so. Ever since the NHS's foundation in the 1940s, it has adapted its shape to the particular administrative and geographical conditions of England, Scotland, Wales and Northern Ireland. But since devolution in 1999, and the transfer of responsibility for healthcare in Scotland, Wales and Northern Ireland to the Scottish Parliament, Welsh Assembly and the Northern Ireland Assembly, the divergence in structure has become more marked. The NHS has also pursued different priorities in each of the four countries.

However, the service's underlying values remain the same. These originate from the 1944 white paper, *A national health service*, which stated that:

> The government want to ensure that in future every man, woman and child can rely on getting all the advice and treatment and care they may need in matters of personal health; that what they shall get shall be the best medical and other facilities available; that their getting these shall not depend on whether they can pay for them or any other factor irrelevant to the real need.

Both society and the health service have altered almost beyond recognition since then, but the NHS still strives to provide a broadly comprehensive service, mostly

One nation – four countries

UK population	(million)	% of total
England	50.1	83.7
Scotland	5.1	8.5
Wales	2.9	4.9
Northern Ireland	1.7	2.9
Total	**59.8**	**100**

Source: Office for National Statistics

Vital statistics: NHS spending per head in the UK 2005/06 (£)

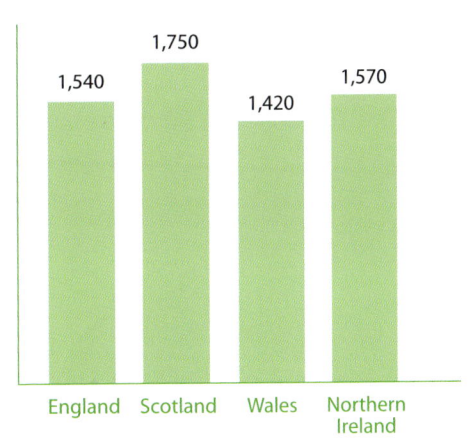

- England: 1,540
- Scotland: 1,750
- Wales: 1,420
- Northern Ireland: 1,570

Sources: DH, Scottish Executive Health Department, Welsh Assembly Government, Northern Ireland DHSSPS

free to all at the point of need. Of course, it has had to move with the times to take advantage of scientific and technological advances, as well as political, social and economic change. Major reform programmes have been under way in all four parts of the UK for the past six years. Certain principles remain common to all four systems:

- The NHS provides a universal service for all, based on clinical need, not ability to pay.
- It provides a comprehensive range of services.
- It strives to shape its services around the needs and preferences of individual patients, their families and their carers.
- The NHS aims to respond to the different needs of different populations.
- It works continuously to improve quality services and to minimise errors.
- It supports and values its staff.
- Public funds for healthcare are devoted solely to NHS patients.
- The NHS works with others to ensure a seamless service for patients.
- It aims to help keep people healthy and work to reduce health inequalities.
- The NHS respects the confidentiality of individual patients and provides open access to information about services, treatment and performance.

However, the Department of Health is consulting on a set of modified principles that would apply to 'all NHS and independent sector providers who sign national model NHS contracts with commissioners' in England, which would further reflect the extent to which the NHS is diverging in different parts of the UK.

What the NHS does: contacts per day (thousands)

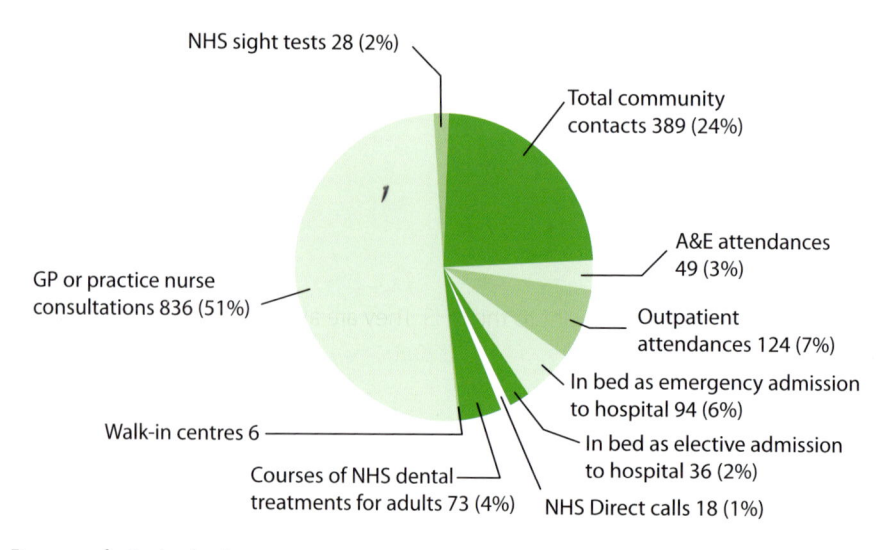

- NHS sight tests 28 (2%)
- Total community contacts 389 (24%)
- A&E attendances 49 (3%)
- GP or practice nurse consultations 836 (51%)
- Outpatient attendances 124 (7%)
- In bed as emergency admission to hospital 94 (6%)
- Walk-in centres 6
- In bed as elective admission to hospital 36 (2%)
- Courses of NHS dental treatments for adults 73 (4%)
- NHS Direct calls 18 (1%)

Figures are for England only.

Source: Department of Health

1

Part 1: the NHS in England
The structure of the NHS in England

Parliament

As the NHS is financed mainly through taxation it relies on Parliament for its funds, and has to account to Parliament for their use through the Secretary of State for Health, the cabinet member responsible for the service. Parliament scrutinises the service through debates, MPs' questions to ministers and select committees. These procedures mean that the Government has to publicly explain and defend its policies for the NHS. The Scottish Parliament (page 162), the Welsh Assembly (page 180) and the Northern Ireland Assembly (page 194) are responsible for oversight of the NHS in their parts of the UK.

Select committees
Three select committees, each comprising backbench MPs representing the major parties, are particularly relevant to the NHS. They are all able to summon ministers, civil servants and NHS employees to give oral or written evidence to their inquiries, usually in public. Their reports are published throughout the parliamentary session.

Health committee
The health committee's role is 'to examine the expenditure, administration and policy of the Department of Health and its associated bodies'. It has a maximum of

11 members. Recent inquiries covered aspects of IT in the NHS and patient and public involvement.

www.parliament.uk

Public accounts committee

The public accounts committee is concerned with ensuring the NHS is operating with economy, efficiency and effectiveness. Its inquiries are based on reports about the service's 'value for money', produced by the Comptroller and Auditor General, who heads the National Audit Office. It aims to draw lessons from past successes and failures that can be applied to future activity. The committee has 16 members, and is traditionally chaired by an Opposition MP.

www.parliament.uk
www.nao.gov.uk

Public administration committee

The public administration committee examines reports from the Health Service Commissioner (better known as the Ombudsman, see page 100). It has 11 members.

www.parliament.uk
www.ombudsman.org.uk

Health ministers

The Department of Health has six ministers: the Secretary of State, four ministers of state and a parliamentary under-secretary of state. The Secretary of State is a member of the cabinet and has overall responsibility for NHS and social care delivery and system reforms, finance and resources and strategic communications. The other ministers each have specific areas of NHS activity assigned to them. The Department for Education and Skills has the lead for children's issues, and the Department for Work and Pensions has the lead for issues affecting older people. Both work closely with the Department of Health.

The Department of Health

The role of the Department of Health (DH) is to support the Government in improving the health and well-being of the population in England. It provides strategic leadership to the NHS and social care organisations, setting their overall direction while deciding and monitoring standards. It negotiates levels of NHS funding with the Treasury, and allocates resources to the health service at large. The DH's 2,224 staff are based in London and Leeds.

The Scottish Executive Health Department (page 164) the Welsh Health and Social Care Department (page 181) and Northern Ireland's Department of Health, Social Services and Public Safety (page 196) provide strategic leadership for the NHS in their parts of the UK.

Further information
Departmental report, DH, May 2006.
Department of Health business plan 2006–07, DH, December 2006.
www.dh.gov.uk

The permanent secretary and NHS chief executive
These two roles were combined in 2000 but then separated again in 2006. The permanent secretary is the DH's most senior civil servant, responsible for the day-to-day running of the department. The NHS chief executive is responsible for the service's management and performance. Both are responsible to the Secretary of State. The chief executive's report to the NHS is published each year and outlines the service's progress towards meeting key objectives. The chief executive also produces a weekly bulletin, e-mailed every Thursday to NHS and council chief executives and directors of social services, containing details of publications, circulars and announcements.

Further information
Chief executive's report to the NHS, DH, June 2006.

Department of Health top management structure

Chief Medical Officer	Permanent Secretary	NHS Chief Executive
Healthcare Quality	Finance and Investment	Commissioning
Programmes	Policy and Strategy	Access
Research and Development	Chief Nursing Officer	Programmes and Performance
Health Improvement	Social Care	Workforce
Health Protection, International Health and Scientific Development	Care Services	Commercial
Regional Public Health Groups/Directors of Public Health	Equality and Human Rights	Connecting for Health/IT
	Communications	
	Departmental Management	
	Arm's-length Bodies Review	

Source: Department of Health

The DH board

The board's role is to provide strategic leadership and help achieve ministers' policy aims. Specifically, it:
- agrees a departmental business plan with annual and longer-term objectives
- sets performance and quality targets
- reviews DH performance
- agrees a framework for corporate governance and holds directors to account
- develops strategy in line with DH values and principles
- ensures DH plans and performance take key stakeholders into account.

The permanent secretary chairs the board, whose members are:
- NHS chief executive
- chief medical officer
- chief nursing officer
- director of finance and investment
- director of policy and strategy
- director general for provider development
- director general of communications
- director general of social care
- director general of IT
- director general of workforce
- commissioning director
- commercial director
- two non-executive directors.

In addition, the national director for social care, the director for equality and human rights and a deputy chief medical officer report directly to the DH board, though they are not members of it.

Chief professional officers

Chief professional officers provide expert knowledge in specialist health and social care disciplines. They comprise:
- chief medical officer
- chief nursing officer
- chief dental officer
- chief health professions officer
- chief pharmaceutical officer
- chief scientific officer.

The chief medical officer (CMO) is the Government's principal medical adviser and the professional head of all medical staff in England. The CMO produces an independent annual report on the state of the nation's health.

National clinical directors

National clinical directors are experts in their field and oversee implementation of national service frameworks. Their roles vary but include chairing taskforces, promoting the work of their specialism, developing clinical networks and advising on clinical quality and governance. They focus on delivering care rather than DH policy. They are:
- national clinical director for emergency access
- national director for mental health
- national director for heart disease
- national director for patients and the public
- national clinical director for primary care
- national director for *Valuing People*, the learning disability strategy
- co-national director for learning disabilities
- national director for older people's services and neurological conditions
- national cancer director
- national clinical director for diabetes
- national clinical director for children
- national director for widening participation in learning
- national director of pandemic influenza preparedness.

Arm's-length bodies

Arm's-length bodies are stand-alone national organisations with executive functions, sponsored by the Department of Health. They vary in size but tend to have boards, employ staff and publish accounts. There are three kinds of ALB:
- executive agencies, such as the Medicines and Healthcare Products Regulatory Agency (see page 215); these are part of the DH and accountable to it
- special health authorities – which provide a service to the whole of England rather than to a local community. They are independent, but can be subject to ministerial direction like other NHS bodies
- non-departmental public bodies, which are set up when ministers want independent advice without direct influence from Whitehall departments.

ALBs are accountable to the DH and sometimes directly to Parliament. They have existed since the NHS was set up in 1948, and numbered 38 by 2004 when the Government announced it was to review and rationalise them, creating six new ones but cutting them to 19 overall by 2008. Their roles will be:
- regulation
- public welfare and standards
- central services to the NHS.

Strategic health authorities

In England, ten strategic health authorities (SHAs) are accountable to the DH for ensuring their local health systems operate effectively. (See later sections for management arrangements in Scotland, page 166; Wales, page 182; and Northern Ireland, page 197.) SHAs are almost coterminous with the Government Offices for the Regions (see page 160). Their main functions are:
- developing strategic partnerships at regional level
- strategic oversight of primary care trusts, especially in assessing capacity and the local supply of healthcare; ensuring competition and contestability, supporting reconfiguration and achieving financial recovery
- helping implement national projects such as Connecting for Health (see page 136)
- helping develop and evaluate national policy
- managing corporate affairs such as communication, reputation management and parliamentary business
- developing organisations and the workforce, including help for NHS trusts to become foundation trusts, and encouraging new providers such as social enterprises
- assessing primary care trusts and managing their performance.

The Office of the Strategic Health Authorities (OSHA) was set up in 2003 to help SHAs work collectively. Its three core functions are:
- providing SHAs with a joint executive
- providing a focal point for their relationships with the DH and other national bodies
- helping them share learning and experience.

The SHAs fund OSHA jointly, and the ten SHA chief executives meet monthly to manage their business through the office.
www.osha.nhs.uk

Strategic health authorities

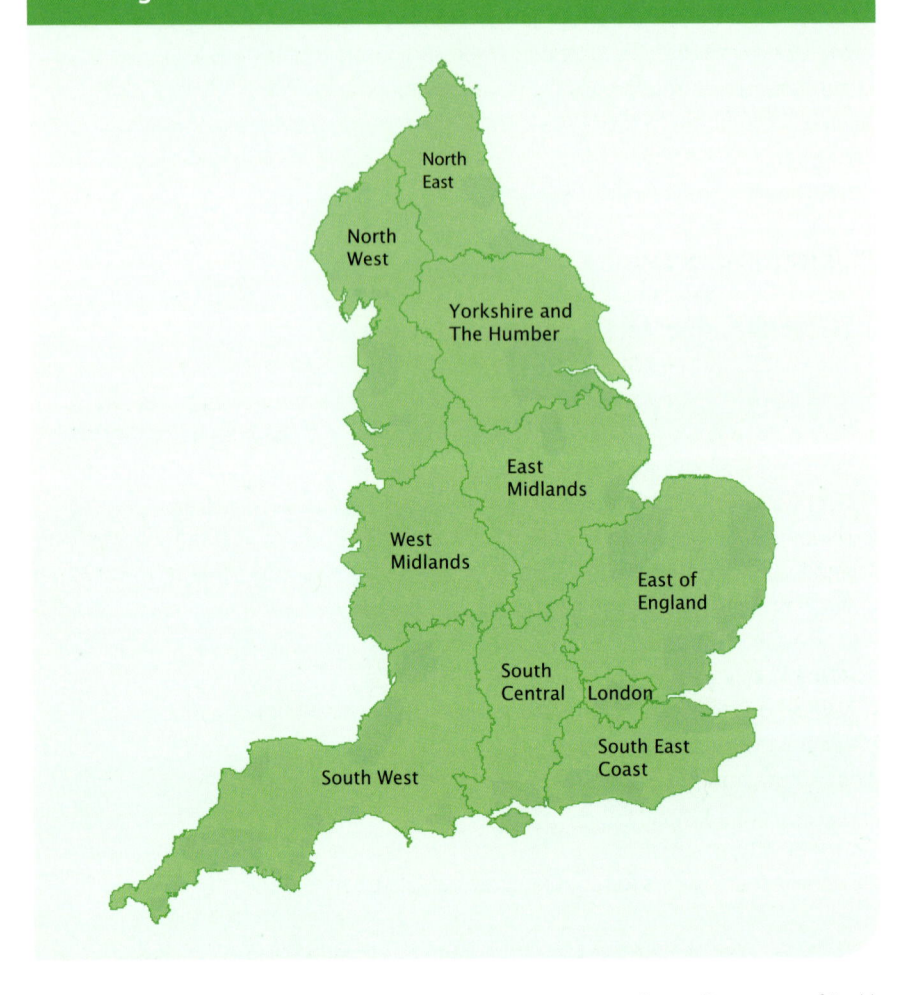

Source: Department of Health

Primary care trusts

In England, primary care trusts (PCTs) are the cornerstone of the NHS locally. Their equivalents in Scotland, community health partnerships, manage primary and community health services, as do Wales's local health boards. Northern Ireland is proposing to create seven local commissioning groups that will be driven by GPs.

PCTs have shared management arrangements where senior management teams cover more than one PCT, albeit with separate board and professional executive committee structures. The 152 PCTs (reconfigured in 2006 from 303) have an average population of 330,000 and are responsible for over 85 per cent of the NHS budget. About 70 per cent of them are coterminous with social services departments.

PCTs' main functions are:
- improving the health of their population – reducing health inequalities in partnership with the local authority; protecting health; emergency planning
- commissioning services – for acute care, by supporting practice-based commissioners (see page 22); for primary care, by retaining full responsibility at PCT level; assessing need, reviewing provision and deciding priorities; designing services; shaping supply through placing contracts; managing demand and performance-managing providers
- directly providing services – where PCTs can show this is in patients' interests and is value for money; a PCT's provider function must be clearly separated from its commissioning function from board-level down.

Further information
Leading edge 20: First steps in planning primary care trust provision, NHS Confederation, November 2006.
Primary care trusts: serving communities, NHS Confederation, 2006.

Contracting
PCTs have four options for providing primary care services.

- They can use the nationally agreed general medical services (GMS) contract (see page 129) to determine the services a GP practice will provide. Revised in 2006, this allows GPs flexibility over the services they offer. It has enabled some to reduce their workload – important in helping the NHS recruit and retain GPs – while others have taken on new services; remuneration is adjusted accordingly. For example, practices can choose to hand over responsibility for evening, weekend and bank holiday services to their local PCT, which must ensure that at least the same level of services continues. Practices have to provide essential services – which means treating sick and terminally ill patients – but can opt out of providing 'additional' services such as child immunisation, maternity and contraceptive services and cervical tests. Most have maintained or expanded the range of services they provide.

- PCTs can use a locally agreed arrangement with practices, the personal medical services (PMS) contract. This enables them to offer salaried appointments to GPs, particularly useful where it has been difficult to recruit and retain them using the GMS contract. PMS contract terms are decided between the PCT and GP to tailor services to local needs. Almost half of GPs now work to PMS contracts.

- Under the alternative provider medical services (APMS) arrangements, PCTs can contract with non-NHS bodies such as voluntary or commercial sector providers to supply primary medical services. They may also contract with NHS secondary care organisations – foundation trusts, NHS trusts or other PCTs – for them to provide primary care services.

- Finally, PCTs can provide services themselves (PCTMS), employing GPs and their practice staff and taking on practice lists and services.

Where PCTs encounter problems securing adequate GP services, the DH insists they 'actively commission additional practices' from diverse suppliers, including the independent sector. 'Change will be driven locally, with local authority input, and co-ordinated nationally in a series of procurement waves', it said in the white paper, *Our health, our care, our say*. It promised to ensure that 'the principles of contestability and value for money are realised under a fair, transparent and consistent process'.

Further information
NHS Primary Care Contracting (employers' web area):
www.primarycarecontracting.nhs.uk

Commissioning

Commissioning is mainly the responsibility of PCTs, delivered through a partnership with general practice (see practice-based commissioning, page 22) and local government. Joint commissioning with local government brings together PCTs and social services for strategic planning and development.

The essential elements of sound commissioning are:
- assessing needs, based on rigorous analysis
- reviewing service provision – identifying gaps and the potential for improving existing services

The organising framework for the health reforms

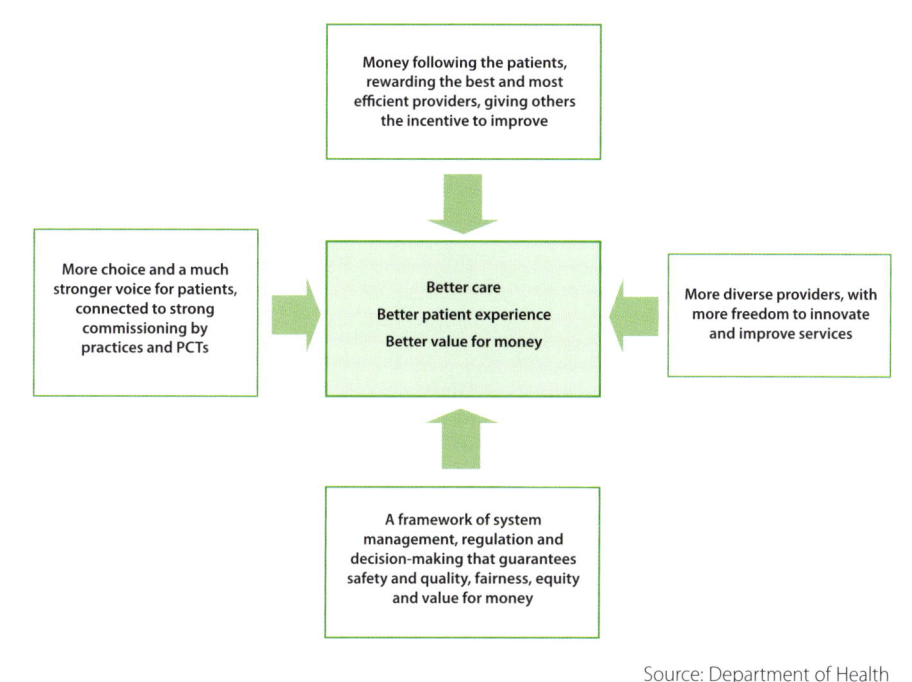

```
                    Money following the patients,
                    rewarding the best and most
                    efficient providers, giving others
                    the incentive to improve
                              ↓
More choice and a much                              More diverse providers, with
stronger voice for patients,   Better care          more freedom to innovate
connected to strong       →  Better patient experience ←  and improve services
commissioning by             Better value for money
practices and PCTs
                              ↑
                    A framework of system
                    management, regulation and
                    decision-making that guarantees
                    safety and quality, fairness, equity
                    and value for money
```

Source: Department of Health

- deciding priorities – the PCT should produce a strategic plan for the health community
- designing services – practices work individually or in groups to develop strategies and service models to improve services
- PCT prospectus – signalling the strategic direction for local services and highlighting commissioning priorities
- shaping the structure of supply – PCTs must be clear about the services and specifications needed, and will agree contracts with local providers within the new national contracting framework
- managing demand and ensuring appropriate access to care – practices and PCTs should establish strategies for the use of care and resources
- clinical decision-making – individual practices and clinicians will undertake individual needs assessments, make referrals and advise patients on choices and treatments

Spotlight on policy: practice-based commissioning

Practice-based commissioning is a reform designed to give GPs and practice nurses more say in how the NHS provides services for patients. Since 2005, GP practices have been able to hold an 'indicative' budget – money their PCT would otherwise control – to spend on secondary services. The intention is that practices will reflect their patients' preferences, leading to greater variety of services from a greater number of providers and more convenience for patients, as well as more efficient use of resources. Practices may combine together to commission services. PCTs continue to be legally responsible for contracting, but practices can keep up to 70 per cent of any savings to reinvest in premises, diagnostic or other equipment, patient services or staff.

The policy is designed to encourage alternative pathways for patients across primary and secondary care. It is also in line with the Government's overarching aims of devolving responsibility and increasing patient choice. By the end of 2006, there were 7,849 practices (93 per cent) taking part in practice-based commissioning, with the Government on target to achieve universal coverage.

Further information
Practice-based commissioning: practical implementation, DH, November 2006.

- managing performance – practices must manage their indicative budget to maximise the benefits from available resources
- patient and public feedback – PCTs are responsible for measuring and reporting on patients' experience.

Further information
Health reform in England: update and commissioning framework, DH, July 2006.

Teaching PCTs

Teaching PCTs (tPCTs), set up mainly in areas of deprivation or where it has been difficult to recruit, are able to offer GPs and other health professionals clinical posts that involve teaching, research or development. They are not confined to traditional teaching activities such as postgraduate clinical training, continuing professional development and lifelong learning, but aim to provide activities that encompass the ethos of learning, development, research, dissemination and good practice. By offering this type of career development, tPCTs hope to attract additional high-quality staff, particularly to deprived areas.

After the 2006 reconfiguration, tPCTs did not automatically keep their teaching status but had to seek approval from their SHA.

NHS trusts

In 2006 there were in England:
- 165 acute trusts
- seven combined acute and community services trusts
- 39 specialist mental health trusts
- two learning disability trusts
- 12 community trusts
- 12 ambulance trusts.

NHS trusts were abolished in Scotland in 2004. Wales has 14, while Northern Ireland is reducing its 18 trusts to five by mid-2007.

NHS trusts earn their income through providing healthcare commissioned by PCTs and practice-based commissioners, as set out in a service level agreement between the organisations. They have a legal duty to break even financially, earn a 6 per cent return on their capital and achieve minimum quality standards. They must work in partnership with other NHS organisations, local authorities and the voluntary sector. Trusts are also obliged to deliver national priorities.

Although strategic health authorities manage their performance, trusts are largely self-governing organisations. Their boards comprise a chair, five non-executive directors and five executives – including the chief executive and usually the medical, nursing and finance directors. NHS trusts employ most of the health service's workforce. The Government intends that all NHS trusts will become foundation trusts by April 2008.

Foundation trusts

Foundation trusts are designed to give greater freedom to NHS organisations, as part of the wider programme of moving from a service controlled nationally to one where standards and inspection are national but delivery and accountability are local. They are unique to the NHS in England.

They are independent public benefit organisations, modelled on co-operatives and mutual societies, but remain part of the NHS – subject to its standards, performance ratings and inspection systems. Foundation trusts are still accountable to Parliament, but local people have a say in running them by becoming members or governors (see page 37).

Monitor, the independent regulator of NHS foundation trusts, authorises NHS trusts applying for foundation status and ensures they comply with the terms of their authorisation. Monitor is accountable to Parliament but independent of the Health Secretary, and has powers to intervene in the running of a foundation trust if it fails to meet standards or breaches the terms of its authorisation. The Healthcare Commission (see page 82) inspects the performance of foundation trusts, as it does all other NHS organisations.

Foundation trusts' main advantages include:
- increased freedom to retain any operating surpluses – for example, from land sales – and access to capital from both the public and private sectors; the amount a foundation trust can borrow will be determined by a formula based on its ability to repay the loan, and governed by the prudential borrowing code set by Monitor
- an obligation to achieve national targets and standards like the rest of the NHS, but freedom to decide how they do this
- not being subject to directions from the Secretary of State
- powers to establish private companies
- the ability to vary staff pay from nationally agreed terms and conditions, although Agenda for Change (see page 128) does apply to foundation trusts
- not being subject to performance management by strategic health authorities and the DH.

There are currently 58 foundation trusts, including the first five mental health trusts. More than 30 others have won the Secretary of State's support to apply for foundation status, and the Government expects up to 100 to be operating by the end of 2007. Foundation trusts are currently responsible for well over a quarter of acute and specialist trust provision, and employ 185,000 staff. Eligibility for foundation trust status was initially restricted to the highest-performing NHS trusts, but the Government has broadened this with the intention that all NHS trusts will be eligible by 2008. It is also exploring the possibility of foundation status for community services managed by PCTs. The Whole Health Community Diagnostic Project is assessing the viability of trusts that have not yet applied for foundation status.

Further information
A short guide to NHS foundation trusts, DH, November 2005.
NHS foundation trusts: report for six-month period to 30 September 2006, Monitor, December 2006.
Review of foundation trusts, Healthcare Commission, July 2005.
Foundation trusts: two years on, Foundation Trust Network, 2006.
NHS foundation trusts ... making a difference, Foundation Trust Network, 2005.
Foundation Trust Network: **www.foundationtrustnetwork.org**
Monitor: **www.regulator-nhsft.gov.uk/index.php**

Care trusts

Care trusts are designed to allow close integration of health and social care. They commission and provide both within a single NHS organisation. (Health and social services have been fully integrated in Northern Ireland since 1972.)

The NHS and a local authority may establish a care trust together where both agree it offers the best way to improve health and social care. NHS and local authority health-related functions are delegated to the trust, not transferred, and the arrangement is voluntary – partners can withdraw. Local authority councillors are members of the care trust's board. Care trusts may be based on either a primary care trust or an NHS trust.

The concept is intended to be flexible enough to allow for a range of models and service configurations, but care trusts are likely to focus on specialist mental health and older people's services. There are currently 12 care trusts. However, there are increasing examples of PCT and adult social care coming together in shared management arrangements, although not always using the care trust organisational mode.

Children's trusts

The Government's long-term aim, as stated in the 2004 green paper, *Every child matters*, is to integrate key children's services within a single organisational focus, the preferred model for which is children's trusts. All areas should have them by 2008. Progress is being evaluated in 35 pathfinder children's trusts.

A children's trust will have the following core features:
- clear short- and long-term objectives
- a children's services director in overall charge of delivering these objectives
- a single planning and commissioning function, supported by pooled budgets.

The trust should involve children and families in putting together a picture of their needs and in designing the services to meet those needs through public, private, voluntary and community providers.

Managed clinical networks

Clinical networks, first developed in Scotland (see page 168) are not statutory bodies but partnerships of all organisations and professionals involved in commissioning, planning and providing a particular service in a geographical area. They form, in effect, virtual organisations, and have the potential to break down barriers between primary, secondary and tertiary care and between health and social care. Good working relationships are crucial to their success, and they need multidisciplinary leadership and management.

Networks help ensure all staff with whom a patient has contact are working to the same protocols and policies – for example, on admission, discharge and transfer; this can ease bed shortages and reduce the need for transferring patients between facilities. By collecting all information relevant to a clinical condition they enable network-wide audit to inform practice and future service developments. They encourage staff to work as one on common issues, and share learning.

Networks are now well developed in cancer care, bringing together commissioners and providers, the voluntary sector and local authorities. There are currently 34 cancer care networks, each serving one to two million people.

Key organisations

NHS Networks
NHS Networks is not so much an organisation as an 'initiative and website to connect leaders and innovators across the NHS with each other and with policy formers – joining networks up across geographies, sectors, professions and government'. Its small team aims to mobilise the expertise and connections of existing networks, and provide logistical support to help them achieve results quickly. Its website is intended to be 'a shop window for networks, and a working tool for networking', where participants can share case studies, exchange information and get in touch with those who run networks and promote good practice. Themes range from human resources through clinical topics to prison health innovation and many more. At the beginning of 2007, 300 networks were registered.
www.networks.nhs.uk

Care Services Improvement Partnership
CSIP raises awareness of national and local initiatives to develop managed local networks in children's and maternity services. It acts as a central point of communication, helping to share information, resources and expertise.
www.csip.org.uk

New providers

The Government declared in *Growing capacity*: 'The NHS cannot remain a monolithic, centrally run monopoly provider. Ideological or institutional boundaries should not stand in the way of better care for NHS patients.'

In order to change the nature and increase the volume of services, it is now an explicit policy to achieve a greater plurality of providers. The Government has said plainly that it wants this to be a permanent development. 'Working with providers from the independent sector and from overseas is not a temporary measure. They will become a permanent feature of the new NHS landscape and will provide NHS services. Different healthcare providers will work to a common ethos, common standards and a common system of inspection.'

By 2008 the Government envisages that the independent sector may provide up to 15 per cent of operations and an increasing number of diagnostic procedures to NHS patients. All independent sector providers must pass the key test of ensuring high standards of care and good value for money.

In addition, the Government is offering help to PCTs to commission primary care services from 'a diverse set of suppliers for communities that have previously been poorly served', according to the white paper, *Our health, our care, our say*. The Government had earlier said it wanted to introduce 'some radically different types of provision' that will 'involve freeing up the entrepreneurialism within primary care and developing new types of provider organisations'. It predicted these would include 'providers who are currently part of the NHS; established independent suppliers such as GPs and their teams, pharmacies and independent hospitals; other parts of the statutory sector; the voluntary sector; and new entrants from the independent, statutory or voluntary sectors'.

Nevertheless, the Secretary of State has said that, 'In the overall scale of the NHS, the independent sector is small beer' – estimating its contribution at 'about 10 per cent of electives and around 1 per cent of the total NHS budget', and adding that, 'this does not herald the end of NHS provision, or the NHS becoming purely a funder and commissioner of services... In primary and community health services, as in acute hospitals, NHS providers will continue to flourish'.

Further information
Creating a level playing field: a fair environment for patient care, NHS Confederation, 2006.
Independent providers ... making a difference in the NHS, NHS Confederation, 2006.
Growing capacity: a new role for external healthcare providers in England, DH, June 2002.
Creating a patient-led NHS – delivering the NHS Improvement Plan, DH, March 2005.

The private sector
Long-established private healthcare providers in the UK have tended to concentrate on secondary care, but with Government encouragement they and new entrants to the market are now looking for opportunities in primary care too. The DH is particularly keen to see more diverse provision in traditionally 'under-doctored' locations. New private sector providers may include the domestic and international providers of diagnostic services, high street retailers or

Vital statistics: NHS spending on non-NHS healthcare

1997/98	£1,108m
1998/99	£1,230m
1999/00	£1,301m
2000/01	£1,549m
2001/02	£1,793m
2002/03	£2,239m
2003/04	£3,316m
2004/05	£3,666m

Source: Department of Health

pharmaceutical companies. Some may wish to concentrate on managing disease-specific pathways such as diabetes, while others may decide to provide discrete services or management infrastructure rather than comprehensive care.

Independent sector treatment centres (ISTCs)

The Government is encouraging independent operators to set up treatment centres (see page 54) to carry out elective surgery and diagnostic tests for NHS patients. Some are partly staffed with overseas clinicians. The intention is that ISTCs will make available additional staff, over and above those already working for the NHS, where extra capacity is needed beyond the increase planned by NHS providers. In the first phase, 29 ISTCs were given the go-ahead, and by 2006 more than 250,000 patients had received treatment or a diagnostic service in an ISTC. A second phase of ISTCs is now being developed, with greater emphasis on integrating them with NHS facilities and on their provision of training.

Further information
Fourth report of session 2005/06: independent sector treatment centres, House of Commons Health Committee, July 2006.
Government's response to the health committee's report on independent sector treatment centres, DH, October 2006.
Independent sector treatment centres: a report from Ken Anderson, commercial director, Department of Health, to the secretary of state for health, DH, February 2006.

The third sector

'Third sector' describes the range of institutions that fall between the public and private sectors. These include small local community and voluntary groups, large and small registered charities, foundations, trusts, co-operatives and social enterprises (see below). They often provide inpatient and outpatient mental health services, sexual health services, drug rehabilitation and palliative care. Many smaller voluntary organisations play a crucial part in community services, particularly for vulnerable and excluded groups, and are often able to bridge divides between statutory services. PCTs are being encouraged to ensure third sector organisations are included in the planning process. The aim is that third sector organisations can become 'equal players' in providing services.

Further information
No excuses. Embrace partnership now. Step towards change! Report of the third sector commissioning task force, DH, July 2006.

Social enterprises

Social enterprises are organisations run on business lines, but which reinvest profits in the community or in service developments. The Government sees encouragement for social enterprise in health and social care as key to reforms. Social enterprises take different forms, and may include co-operatives, trusts or community interest companies. They are estimated to number at least 55,000, have a combined turnover of £27 billion a year and account for 1 per cent of GDP. Social enterprises involve patients and staff in designing and delivering services, improving quality and tailoring services to meet patients' needs. Many feature partnerships with third sector organisations (see above).

The DH's social enterprise unit is identifying 'pathfinder' social enterprises that will lead the way in providing innovative services. A social enterprise fund is being established to help with set-up costs.

Spotlight on policy: promoting NHS services

With a greater diversity of providers competing to supply services to NHS patients, the DH has recently consulted healthcare organisations on a code of practice for promoting NHS services. This is based on three principles:
- information for patients should not be misleading, inaccurate, unfair or offensive
- the NHS's reputation should be protected
- the amount of public money spent on advertising and promotion should not be excessive.

Contracts between PCTs and providers would automatically include signing up to the code.

Further information
Code of practice for promotion of NHS services, DH, November 2006.

Further information
Social Enterprise Coalition **www.socialenterprise.org.uk**

Overseas clinical teams
The NHS sometimes recruits overseas clinical teams to work in concentrated bursts to supplement capacity in existing organisations, especially in ophthalmics and orthopaedics, where waiting lists have been longest. The scheme aims to use spare capacity in overseas healthcare systems, and seeks to avoid undermining the systems of developing countries. In most cases it is based on short periods of activity using rotating teams – several sessions over a few days or a stay of a few weeks – because the clinical staff continue to practise overseas. Teams vary in size from a handful of clinicians to a large clinical team, including full theatre and support staff. They have been recruited from France, Germany, Belgium, South Africa, Spain and Scandinavia. The NHS welcomes enquiries from any country.

Overseas treatment for NHS patients
There is no earmarked central budget for the overseas treatment of NHS patients. PCTs must decide on the strength of the case and available options whether to

refer patients abroad. They must ensure high quality and value for money, and arrange follow-up care to cope with any complications once patients have returned to the UK. Patients will only travel if that is what they want and after a full clinical assessment shows it meets their needs. Lead commissioning arrangements with Guy's and St Thomas' Trust have been set up to help PCTs wishing to refer patients overseas. About 1,200 UK patients are treated abroad every year.

The role of boards

Duties and responsibilities
The roles and responsibilities of NHS boards are broadly the same throughout the UK. They take corporate responsibility for their organisation's strategies and actions.

Boards generally consist of five executives (including the chief executive and finance director) and five non-executives plus a chair. The chair and non-executives are lay people drawn from the local community, and are accountable to the Secretary of State.

A board's main duties are:
- collective responsibility for adding value to the organisation by promoting its success through direction and supervision of its affairs
- providing active leadership within a framework of prudent and effective controls which enable risk to be assessed and managed
- setting the organisation's strategic aims, ensuring the necessary financial and human resources are in place for it to meet its objectives and reviewing management performance
- setting and maintaining the organisation's values and standards, while ensuring its obligations to patients, the local community and the Secretary of State are understood and met.

Legally, there is no distinction between the board duties of executive and non-executive directors: they both share responsibility for the organisation's direction and control. The board is expected to bring about change by making best use of all its resources – financial, staffing, physical infrastructure and knowledge – and working with staff and partner organisations to meet the public's and patients' expectations. As leaders, board members are expected to understand opportunities for improving services and motivate others to bring them about.

Spotlight on policy: cross-border healthcare

The European Commission will publish proposals in 2007 on the principles governing cross-border healthcare in the European Union. Cross-border care is a growing trend, particularly for countries in mainland Europe. Test cases in the European Court of Justice brought by patients seeking reimbursement for cross-border care, or by health systems attempting to restrict treatment of non-residents, have driven developments.

Rulings have created an ambiguous situation, defending both citizens' right to travel and the system's ability to defend financial stability. The court has also stipulated that provisions in the EU's founding Treaty of Rome on free movement of goods and services apply to healthcare regardless of how it is organised or financed – and the court has confirmed this is so even for a tax-funded system like the NHS.

As a result, citizens lack clarity about their entitlement to healthcare abroad or how they might go about identifying, comparing and choosing providers. Member states lack clarity about how they can regulate and plan their systems without creating unjustified obstacles to free movement.

Few UK patients travel abroad for healthcare, given the geographical and language disincentives to do so (though their cases are often well publicised when they do). As NHS waiting times fall, even fewer may travel in future. But as the EC points out, many are interested in cross-border care in principle and would benefit from more information about options in other EU states.

Further information
Consultation 24: The European Commission's public consultation on cross-border healthcare, NHS Confederation, November 2006.

Boards make plans to achieve the Government's objectives for healthcare, guided by the targets and delivery dates in the priorities and planning framework as well as the detailed objectives in the NHS Plan and national service frameworks. Boards have scope to pace their plans to reflect local circumstances, and have a large say over how to achieve them. All boards sign off an annual business plan setting out the year's objectives, and it is the whole board's function to ensure progress.

NHS boards are obliged to ensure their organisations have an ethos and culture of public service that reflects and respects public expectation. The need for public accountability means boards must conduct business in an open and transparent way that commands public confidence. Their meetings are open to the public, and should be understandable to the public.

Further information
Governing the NHS: a guide for boards, DH and NHS Appointments Commission, June 2003.
Effective boards in the NHS? A study of their behaviour and culture, NHS Confederation, 2005.

The chair
As identified by the Higgs Report and modified to reflect the NHS, a chair's main role is:
- leadership of the board, ensuring its effectiveness in all aspects of its role and setting its agenda
- ensuring provision of accurate, timely and clear information to directors
- ensuring effective communication with staff, patients and the public
- arranging regular evaluation of the board's performance, its committees and individual directors
- helping non-executive directors contribute effectively and ensuring constructive relations between executive and non-executive directors.

Chairs are expected to work up to three days a week. In general, a strong correlation exists between the quality of the chair's and chief executive's leadership and the organisation's success. Where an organisation is not delivering, questions can legitimately be asked about the quality of the board leadership.

Non-executive directors

In 2003 the Higgs Report laid out the responsibilities and expectations of non-executives. Although the report was commissioned by the Department of Trade and Industry and the Treasury to look at commercial enterprises, its principles are relevant to all NHS boards.

Non-executives should:
- constructively challenge and contribute to developing strategy, scrutinise managers' performance in meeting objectives and monitor the reporting of performance
- satisfy themselves that financial information is accurate and that financial controls and risk management are robust
- be responsible for deciding executive directors' pay, as well as have a prime role in appointing – and where necessary, removing – senior managers and in succession planning
- ensure the board acts in the public's best interests and is fully accountable to it for the organisation's services and the public funds it uses.

There are about 3,500 chairs and non-executives in NHS organisations in England, excluding foundation trusts. About 1,000 appointments are made each year. Women make up 46 per cent of non-executives, while people from black and minority ethnic groups account for 6 per cent of chairs and non-executives. Non-executives work two-and-a-half days a month and are paid £5,800 a year in NHS trusts and £7,500 a year in SHAs and PCTs. Audit committee chairs in SHAs and PCTs receive an extra £5,000 a year. Chairs work three-and-a-half days a week and are paid between £17,545 and £22,235 a year in NHS trusts, between £30,000 and £40,000 in PCTs and between £40,000 and £60,000 in SHAs, with the London SHA chair receiving £60,000. Foundation trusts set their own rates, which are generally much higher than other NHS organisations.

Further information
Survey of NHS chairs and non-executives, Appointments Commission, 2005.
Review of the roles and effectiveness of non-executive directors (Higgs Report), DTI, January 2003.
Briefing 81: The Higgs Report into the role of non-executive directors, NHS Confederation, May 2003.

The chief executive

The chief executive is responsible for ensuring the board is empowered to govern the organisation and that its objectives are accomplished through effective and properly controlled executive action. A chief executive's main responsibilities are:
- leadership
- delivery planning
- performance management
- governance
- accountability.

Board committees

NHS boards may delegate some of their powers to formally constituted committees. Some are set up to advise the board on a permanent basis, such as the:
- audit committee
- remuneration and terms of service committee
- clinical governance committee
- risk management committee.

PCT boards and PECs

Like other NHS organisations, PCTs are overseen by a board consisting of a lay chair and a majority of non-executives, although they must also include a director of public health. In addition, to reflect the importance of clinical leadership in PCTs, each has a professional executive committee (PEC) with up to 18 members, who may include GPs, nurses, allied health professionals, dentists, pharmacists, optometrists and consultants.

Following PCT reconfiguration and the advent of practice-based commissioning, PECs' future roles, membership and support needs were reviewed and a consultation document published. The DH will issue guidance on the future function of PECs during 2007.

Further information
Consultation on a review of PCTs' professional executive committees, DH, November 2006.
Consultation 23: The future of the professional executive committee, NHS Confederation, October 2006.

Foundation trust boards

Foundation trusts have distinctive governance arrangements to reflect their freedom from central control. Staff, patients and local people are eligible to become 'members' of the trust. Membership entitles them to vote at elections for the board of governors and to stand for election to the board. Members will receive care and treatment at the hospital on exactly the same basis as anyone else. The DH says foundation trusts had recruited 614,000 members by the end of 2006.

The board of governors includes those elected by the trust members and staff, as well as people appointed by PCTs and local authorities. Its role is to advise the board of directors on its forward plans. Foundation trusts had recruited 1,000 governors, including patients, members of the public, staff and representatives from PCTs, universities and voluntary organisations, by the end of 2006.

Each foundation trust has a board of directors made up of non-executives appointed by the governors and executive directors appointed by the non-executives, similar to other NHS organisations. This board is responsible for managing the foundation trust, including its day-to-day operation and forward business plan.

Board of directors' meetings concern the trust's operational business, with board of governors' meetings focusing more on members' needs and ensuring local communities can contribute to decision-making.

Further information

NHS foundation trusts – a guide to developing governance arrangements, DH, September 2004.
New voices, new accountabilities: a guide to foundation trust wider governance, Foundation Trust Network, August 2005.

Key organisation: Appointments Commission

The Appointments Commission specialises in the recruitment, training and appraisal of people for board-level public appointments to NHS bodies, ministerial advisory bodies and other quangos in England. It recruits up to 1,000 people every year through open recruitment campaigns, advertised in local papers. Shortlisted candidates are interviewed by panels that include an independent assessor.

The Commission consists of a chair, a chief executive and eight regional commissioners. It has 45 staff based in London and Leeds, with several regional training facilitators around the country. The commission's board meets monthly to consider panel recommendations and make appointments.

Set up in 2001 following the NHS Plan, the Commission aims to ensure all appointments are made on merit and follow an open, transparent and fair process. Before it existed, health ministers were responsible for appointing all non-executive directors.

The Commission's role does not end once an appointment has been made. Chairs and non-executives look to the regional commissioners for mentoring and support. The Commission ensures that chairs and non-executives receive proper induction and training in their roles, providing 4,000 training places a year.

Further information
Governing the NHS: a guide for NHS boards, DH/NHS Appointments Commission, June 2003.
www.appointments.org.uk

2
Where care is delivered

Primary care

Primary care is where 90 per cent of NHS patients receive their treatment and over 300 million consultations take place every year in England alone. Advances in healthcare, especially in diagnostics and minor surgery, mean many more treatments once carried out in hospital can be performed within primary care – a rapidly growing trend convenient for patients and of benefit to the system as a whole. Over 5 million people in England live more than ten miles from their nearest hospital.

A wide range of staff work in primary care in England. In 2005 there were:
- 35,302 GPs
- 22,904 practice nurses
- 89,190 practice staff, including practice managers, receptionists, IT support and notes summarisers, physiotherapists, podiatrists, counsellors, phlebotomists and healthcare assistants.

Most GP practices are independent contractors and are run as partnerships, although some salaried GPs are employed by primary care trusts, while specialist companies run some practices.

Key text: *Our health, our care, our say*

This white paper sets out the Government's vision for more effective health and social care services outside hospital. Published in January 2006, halfway through the ten-year programme begun with the NHS Plan, its aim is to focus the health service's increased capacity on more 'personalised' care. It built on major public consultation held at five events across England during 2005. The white paper calls for closer integration between health and social services, better access to GPs, improved care for people with long-term conditions and further effort to combat health inequalities.

Its main points include:
- an improved role for community hospitals
- a timetable for more outpatient appointments to be held in primary care
- patients to be allowed to register with practices near to their workplace or home
- extended practice opening times to meet patients' needs
- integration of health and social care planning cycles
- a single complaints procedure across health and social care
- 'NHS Life Check' to assess people's lifestyle risks and target health advice
- 'information prescriptions' for people with long-term conditions
- an urgent-care strategy to improve access to emergency care
- improvements in end-of-life care
- rapid access to sexual health services
- more choice for women in maternity care
- a commitment to close campus-based provision for adults with learning disabilities
- pilot schemes for direct access to allied health professionals.

During 2006, 30 care-closer-to-home pilot sites were launched to assess how consultants, GPs and nurses can provide minor operations and diagnostic tests in urology, ENT, dermatology, orthopaedics, gynaecology and general surgery closer to patients' homes. The DH has also set aside £750 million to develop a new generation of community hospitals and health centres, the first four of which have been approved.

Key text: *Our health, our care, our say* continued

Further information
Our health, our care, our say: making it happen, DH, October 2006.
Briefing 128: Our health, our care, our say – a new direction for community services, NHS Confederation, February 2006.

Supersurgeries

The GP surgery is the focus of most primary care and the source of ever wider-ranging services. The NHS Plan described a vision of the GP surgery of the future:

> Many GPs will be working in teams from modern multi-purpose premises alongside nurses, pharmacists, dentists, therapists, opticians, midwives and social care staff. Nurses will have new opportunities, and some GPs will tend to specialise in treating different conditions. The consulting room will become the place where appointments for outpatients and operations are booked, test results received and more diagnosis carried out using video and tele-links to hospital specialists. An increasing number of consultants will take outpatient sessions in local primary care centres.

PCTs are being encouraged to consider setting up one-stop health centres, which bring services such as GPs, health visitors, dentists, a pharmacy, a cardiology clinic, x-ray facilities, optometry services, Surestart and a healthy living café under one roof. By 2008, the DH estimates, 750 one-stop health centres will have been built since 2001.

Practitioners with a special interest

Primary care services are expanding by developing the role of practitioners with special interests.

GPs with a special interest (GPSIs) have additional training and expertise which enables them to provide a clinical service beyond the scope of normal general practice, undertake advanced procedures or develop services. They take referrals from colleagues for conditions in specialties such as ophthalmology, orthopaedics, dermatology and ear, nose and throat surgery, or undertake diagnostic procedures such as endoscopy. GPSIs do not offer a full consultant service, replace consultants or interfere with access to consultants by local GPs. Typically they undertake two sessions a week in their specialty.

GPSIs can increase the capacity of primary care to undertake outpatient appointments, reduce patient waiting times, provide a more convenient service and help to free consultant time in secondary care. Over 1,200 GPSIs are currently practising.

Initially, emphasis was on developing GPs and nurses with special interests, but allied health professionals have now been included. The DH's Wider Range of Services in Primary Care programme is focused on developing the role of PSIs to undertake outpatient appointments and ensuring primary care facilities can accommodate these additional services.

Further information
GPs with a special interest **www.gpwsi.org.uk**

Walk-in centres

Walk-in centres provide fast access to advice and treatment for minor ailments and injuries without an appointment. By May 2006 there were 75 throughout England with expansion planned up to 89, including seven instant-access GP-led centres for commuters, commissioned from the independent sector. The first opened at Manchester Piccadilly Station in 2005.

Walk-in centres are open seven days a week, from early morning until late evening, and offer assessment by an experienced NHS nurse as well as information on out-of-hours GP, dental and local pharmacy services. In addition to providing a core service, the centres are helping improve access for groups with particular needs, including young people, homeless people, students, refugees and asylum seekers.

The centres saw more than 2.5 million attendances in 2005/06, with an average of 101 a day. Visits increased by 442,000 (21 per cent) in the year to September 2006. As walk-in centres develop, they will offer independent prescribing by nurses and access to GP services so that more patients will receive treatment and prescriptions without having to go to their own practice.

Greater use of new services convenient to patients

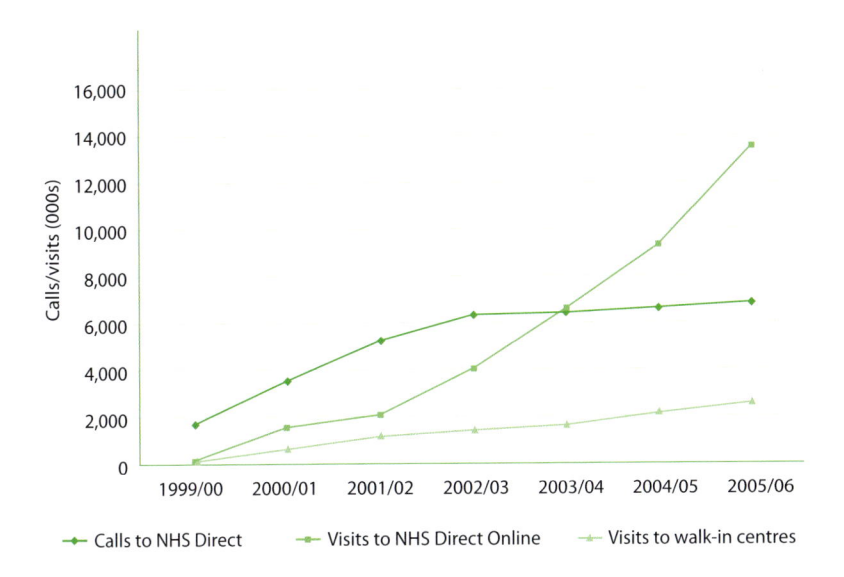

[Chart showing Calls/visits (000s) from 1999/00 to 2005/06, with three lines: Calls to NHS Direct, Visits to NHS Direct Online, Visits to walk-in centres]

Source: NHS chief executive's report June 2006, Department of Health

NHS Direct

NHS Direct is a 24-hour telephone health advice and information service staffed by nurses. It provides callers to its helpline with information on what to do if they or their family are feeling ill, advice on particular health conditions, details of local healthcare services, such as doctors, dentists or late-night pharmacies, as well as self-help and support organisations. Staff use a computer-based decision-support system to suggest the best course of action, and can pass calls directly to emergency services; about 3 per cent of calls are emergencies.

Launched in 1998, NHS Direct handles over half a million calls every month and has served more than 36 million callers in total. During 2004/05, 18 million copies of the NHS Direct self-help guide were delivered to households in England. NHS Direct's phone number provides a single point of access for out-of-hours care and handles all low-priority 999 ambulance calls. The top ten symptoms people call about are fever, abdominal pains, vomiting, rash, cough, diarrhoea, headache, cold or flu, toothache and chest pain.

PCTs are responsible for commissioning NHS Direct services. Formerly a special health authority, NHS Direct became an NHS trust in April 2007.

NHS Direct is piloting NHS Health Direct, proposed in the *Choosing health* white paper (see page 152) as an information service based on the internet, digital television and mobile phones. It is hoped to launch the service nationally in 2008. Plans include:
- a personal health assessment tool
- information on local health improvement services and opportunities
- content on major healthy lifestyle issues
- content generated by users, such as chat rooms, forums and blogs
- personal updates via e-mail and text messages.

NHS Direct in England and Wales operate from the same telephone number – 0845 4647 – while Scotland's information service is called NHS 24 and uses 08454 242424.

NHS Direct Online

NHS Direct Online (**www.nhsdirect.nhs.uk**) is an interactive website that provides:
- a self-help guide to treating common problems at home
- a 'body key' to identify symptoms
- a health encyclopaedia with over 400 topics
- personal responses to specific requests for information
- a searchable database of hospitals and community health services, GPs, dentists, opticians and pharmacies.

The HealthSpace facility offers patients a secure place on NHS Direct Online where, for example, they can record personal health details and make them available to their GP. It provides a secure portal through which to access Choose and Book and electronic transfer of prescriptions.

Visits to NHS Direct Online numbered 13.5 million in 2005/06.

NHS Direct Interactive

NHS Direct Interactive is a health information service for the interactive area on digital TV, including Freeview. It does not broadcast programmes, but its 3,000 pages of content – available in 16 languages – include a health encyclopaedia, advice on diet, exercise, sexual health and smoking cessation, video clips on a range of health topics, a directory of local NHS services plus tips on using the NHS. Users can search for details of their nearest doctors, dentists, pharmacies and opticians by inputting their postcode details. Pilot projects showed that health information on digital TV could reach a wide audience, particularly parts of the population hard to reach through other means, such as people on low incomes, who may not have access to the internet. NHS Direct Interactive can also be viewed on the web (**www.nhsdirect.tv**).

Dental services

Policy on dental services has lagged behind other health sectors. Dentists' commitment to the NHS has waned, leading to problems for many people seeking dental care: numbers of dentists have fallen by about 4 per cent since a new contract was introduced in April 2006, although those remaining do less private and more NHS work. About two-thirds of adults visit their dentist regularly, the rest attending only when they have trouble. Many practices offer a mixture of private and NHS care that can be confusing for patients.

Since 2006, the £1.6 billion budget for primary care dental services has been devolved to PCTs. This covers surgery salaries and expenses instead of the piecework pay system set up when the NHS was founded. Surgeries are being encouraged to broaden their range of services. For the first time, England's 20,890 primary care dentists will be able to focus on prevention and health promotion, as well as treatment within their NHS contracts, and spend more time with patients.

In addition, the Government recruited 1,453 more dentists in 2005, 743 of them from abroad. It has also created 170 extra undergraduate dental training places in England, a 25 per cent increase. A fourfold increase to 200 training places for dental therapists is also underway. Funding for NHS dentistry has risen by almost 20 per cent. In the year to October 2005, an additional 700,000 people in England registered with a dentist.

Further information
NHS Dentistry: delivering change – report by the Chief Dental Officer (England), DH, July 2004.
Choosing better oral health: an oral health plan for England, DH, November 2005.

Community pharmacies

Britain's 10,000 high street pharmacies are visited by 6 million people every day and employ 73 per cent of pharmacists. They increasingly offer services traditionally available only at GPs' surgeries. The pharmacy contract introduced in 2005 aims to improve the range and quality of services of the community pharmacy and integrate it more into the NHS. It defines three tiers of service:

- Essential services must be provided by all community pharmacists. They include dispensing, disposal of medication and support for self-care.
- Advanced services require the pharmacist to have accreditation and/or their premises to meet certain standards. So far, medicines use review and prescription intervention fall in this category.
- Enhanced services are commissioned locally by PCTs. Examples include minor ailment schemes and smoking-cessation services.

Many pharmacies now offer new services such as:
- repeat prescribing, so that patients can get up to a year's supply of medicines without having to revisit their GP
- clinics for people with conditions such as diabetes, high blood pressure or high cholesterol
- signposting other health and social care services and supporting self-care consultation areas.

Since the Government relaxed the entry regulations for retail pharmacy services, a recent review found that more than twice as many pharmacies opened in 2005/06 than in any year since 1992, and that 99 per cent of people can get to a pharmacy by car, walking or public transport within 20 minutes.

Further information
The new contractual framework for community pharmacy, DH, October 2004.
The new community pharmacy framework: moving to implementation, NHS Confederation, December 2004.
Review of progress on reforms to the 'control of entry' system for NHS pharmaceutical contractors – report, DH, January 2007.

Opticians

There are three kinds of registered optician:

Optometrists – or ophthalmic opticians – carry out eye tests, look for signs of eye disease and prescribe and fit glasses and contact lenses. They are graduates who have undertaken a three- or four-year degree in optometry, then spent at least a year in supervised practice before taking professional exams leading to registration with the General Optical Council.

Dispensing opticians fit and sell glasses, and interpret prescriptions, but do not test eyes. Some dispense low-vision aids, and some are qualified to fit contact lenses under instruction from an optometrist.

Ophthalmic medical practitioners are doctors specialising in eyes and eye care. They work to the same terms of service as optometrists.

In addition, ophthalmologists are doctors specialising in eye diseases and most perform eye surgery. They usually work in hospital eye departments. Orthoptists treat disorders of binocular vision, and work in eye departments under the supervision of ophthalmologists. They may also undertake visual screening of children in the community.

Optometrists are independent contractors. Some have specialist skills – for example, in contact lenses, low vision or paediatrics – and can treat patients who would otherwise have to be seen in hospital. Most practices have much of the equipment found in ophthalmology clinics.

Under co-management, or shared care, optometrists working to an agreed protocol undertake specified clinical procedures designed to relieve GPs and the hospital eye service, as well as move patient care into the community. This may cover conditions such as glaucoma, diabetes, cataracts and minor acute eye problems. Optometrists are currently pressing for independent and supplementary prescribing rights.

PCTs are responsible for managing optometrists' contracts. Some employ optometric advisers to provide guidance on issues such as service development, new techniques and treatments, interpreting regulations, investigating complaints and audit.

The recent general optical service review assessed how eye-care services are currently provided and found potential for eye-care professionals in primary care to work alongside hospitals in developing more responsive services for patients with eye conditions such as glaucoma. It also identified scope for greater collaboration between the NHS, social care and the third sector in providing integrated services for patients with low-vision problems and in taking wider action to improve eye health.

Further information
General ophthalmic services review: findings in relation to the framework for primary ophthalmic services, the position of dispensing opticians in relation to the NHS, local optical committees, and the administration of general ophthalmic services payments, DH, January 2007.

Community health services

A range of other health services is provided in the community by a variety of staff and organisations.

Community nurses – who include district nurses with a postgraduate qualification, registered nurses and nursing assistants. More than half the patients they see will be aged over 75. About half their work comes from GP referrals and a quarter from hospital staff; patients and carers can also refer themselves.

Community matrons – as experienced nurses, community matrons use case management techniques with patients who make intensive use of healthcare, to help them remain at home longer.

Health visitors – qualified nurses or midwives with additional training and experience in child health, health promotion and education. Much of their work is with mothers and babies using a child-centred, family-focused approach, although they do provide more general health advice to people of all ages. Their support staff include nursery nurses and healthcare assistants, who focus on less complex family support and parenting skills.

Specialist nurses – with expertise in stoma care, continence services, palliative care and support for people with long-term conditions.

Key organisation: Future Healthcare Network

The FHN comprises over 50 trusts and PCTs involved in major investment projects, mainly healthcare-related buildings but also equipment and technology. Part of the NHS Confederation, the FHN's work programme covers strategic planning across the health and care system, design and procurement. Its members network among themselves and with leading external experts, identify best practice, learn from historical and comparative experience and develop innovative models of service development. The FHN brings this leading-edge thinking and practice together to influence national policy and guidance.
www.fhn.org.uk

School nursing – providing support and advice to schools on health issues, a role which has evolved considerably in recent years.

Community dentistry and dental public health – providing services to schools and people who are difficult to treat.

Podiatry – foot care for elderly people or those with diabetes, gait or lower limb problems. Independent contractors provide much of this care. More than half the service is for people aged over 65.

Physiotherapy – sometimes provided by GPs or hospitals in a community setting, with emphasis on rehabilitation.

Occupational therapy – providing advice, aids and adaptations. Some staff specialise in adults, some in children. The service is often provided by other agencies, such as local government, although in some cases the NHS provides local authority OT services.

Speech and language therapy – services for children and adults who have difficulty with communicating, eating, drinking or swallowing.

Clinical psychology – often provided by specialist mental health trusts, although more than 40 per cent of referrals come from general practice.

Midwives – generally attached to hospitals, but working in community settings.

Family planning services – may cover sexual health problems as well as contraception, vasectomy and termination clinics and specialist clinics for young people.

Community rehabilitation – often for stroke or cardiac conditions. Services may be delivered by specialist teams in the patient's home or by combining intermediate care (see below) or community hospital care with home care.

Community hospitals – their focus varies but may include minor injuries, diagnostic and screening services, minor surgery and outpatient clinics. Some offer intermediate care or rehabilitation services. Some are staffed exclusively by nurses supported by local GPs, others by hospital outreach services. In the *Our health, our care, our say* white paper, the Government announced its intention to develop 'a new generation of modern NHS community hospitals'. These will provide diagnostics, day surgery and outpatient facilities. The Government is making available £750 million for this over five years.

Further information
Community Hospitals Association **www.communityhospitals.org.uk**

Intermediate care

Intermediate care is a vital component of the programme to improve the health and well-being of older people and raise the quality of services they receive. Older people are the main users of the NHS: although they make up about a fifth of the population, they occupy two-thirds of hospital beds, and are three times more likely to be admitted to hospital.

Intermediate care comprises a range of services to promote faster recovery from illness, prevent unnecessary hospital admission, support timely discharge from hospital and maximise a patient's ability to live independently. These services may include:

Key texts

National Service Framework for long-term conditions
More than 17.5 million people in the UK suffer from a long-term condition such as diabetes, asthma or arthritis. This NSF sets 11 quality requirements to transform the way health and social care services support people with long-term neurological conditions to live as independently as possible – although much of the guidance applies to anyone with a long-term condition. The requirements include early recognition, prompt diagnosis and treatment, early and specialist rehabilitation, providing equipment and accommodation and supporting family and carers. They are to be fully implemented by 2015. The NSF was published in March 2005.

Supporting people with long-term conditions. An NHS and social care model to support local innovation and integration
Under this model, published in January 2005, health and social care organisations must assign 'community matrons' to the most vulnerable patients with complex multiple long-term conditions to monitor their condition, anticipate any problems and co-ordinate their care. Multi-professional teams will identify all people with a single serious long-term illness, assess their needs as early as possible and provide proactive care before their condition deteriorates. Everyone with a long-term condition will be educated about their health and encouraged to manage their own care more effectively.

- rapid-response teams
- hospital-at-home schemes
- supported-discharge teams
- nurse-led facilities in acute or community settings
- council-run or independent residential rehabilitation.

By its nature, intermediate care is not the preserve of any single profession, organisation or sector. It includes health and social care as well as housing, and relies on partnerships between organisations and professions: health and social care jointly fund 5,000 intermediate care beds. It has developed enormously in recent years and is on the brink of being recognised as a mainstream service. But as its origins pre-date now established policy directions, intermediate care has evolved in many parts of the country through locally led initiatives in response to local service pressures. This has produced a wide diversity of models.

Secondary care

The changing role of hospitals

Acute hospitals have always dominated healthcare spending and provision. But they will be unable to avoid fundamental change in the next five to ten years. As the *Our health, our care, our say* white paper says: 'In future, far more care will be provided in more local and convenient settings. People want this, and changes in technology and clinical practice are making it safer and more feasible.' Meanwhile, patient choice, payment by results and practice-based commissioning will shift the balance of power between organisations, stimulating further change – especially as value for money will become ever more important with the slowdown in spending increases after 2008.

The DH is working with six specialties in 20 to 30 demonstration sites to develop models of providing care 'closer to home'. The specialties are:
- ear, nose and throat
- trauma and orthopaedics
- dermatology
- urology
- gynaecology
- general surgery.

In addition, the two national clinical directors for emergency care and for heart disease and stroke have argued for changes to how their services are delivered. They point out that traditional hospital accident and emergency departments are no longer the only – or even the most – appropriate place to treat such conditions, despite recent major improvements to A&E departments.

Local hospitals are likely to remain important, but rather than working in isolation will have to work much more in collaboration with other providers and each other as part of 'multi-hospital networks of care'. Rather than exercising local monopolies, hospitals will need to promote competition and choice.

Vital statistics: NHS operations in 2005/06

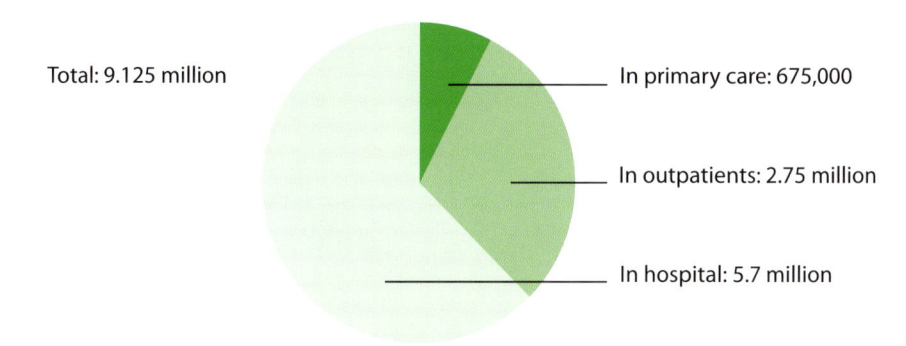

Total: 9.125 million

In primary care: 675,000

In outpatients: 2.75 million

In hospital: 5.7 million

Source: The Information Centre

In 2006 the DH commissioned Sir Ian Carruthers to review the process of reconfiguring services. He concluded: 'Change can all too frequently lead to a loss of public confidence in service providers if the process is not managed carefully, and stakeholders are not fully engaged as early as possible… It must not be change for the sake of change.'

His main recommendations included:
- reasons for change need to be clear and well articulated, and cases for change need to be stronger than they have sometimes been in the past
- clinicians, staff and their representatives need to be more involved in developing proposals locally, regionally and nationally
- coherent and co-ordinated local proposals are essential, with PCTs at the centre of major service change
- communications need to be strengthened, with consultation documents in plain English containing specific and relevant information
- new leadership teams need to review inherited schemes and assure the DH they are fit for purpose.

Further information
Service improvement: quality assurance of major changes to service provision, DH, February 2007.
Briefing 131: Strengthening local services – the future of the acute hospital, NHS Confederation, April 2006.
Emergency access – clinical case for change: report by Sir George Alberti, the national director for emergency access, DH, December 2006.

Mending hearts and brains – clinical case for change: report by Professor Roger Boyle, national director for heart disease and stroke, DH, December 2006.
The future of acute care, Andy Black, NHS Confederation, January 2006.
Keeping the NHS local: a new direction of travel, DH, February 2003.

Treatment centres

Treatment centres are units that carry out planned surgery and treatment in areas that have traditionally had the longest waiting times, separating them from unplanned care and so lessening the risk that operations have to be cancelled. The Government has looked to them to create innovation, increase productivity and rapidly expand capacity. They are developing new staff roles, including perioperative specialist practitioners, advanced nurse practitioners/advisers and healthcare assistant technicians in radiology, ophthalmology and surgery.

Key organisation: Independent Reconfiguration Panel

The IRP advises the Secretary of State on proposals for changes to NHS services that have been contested locally. It also offers support and advice to the NHS, local authorities and others on NHS reconfiguration issues.

The local authority overview and scrutiny committee may refer a proposal if it is not satisfied:
- with the content of the consultation or the time allowed
- with the reasons given for not carrying out consultation
- that the proposal is in the interests of the health service locally.

Although the IRP is a last resort when all other options for local resolution have been fully explored, it welcomes early informal contact in order to avoid formal referral if possible. Once a case is accepted for the IRP to consider, the chair agrees any specific terms of reference and a timetable for reporting. The chair will normally appoint a sub-group of three (one health professional, one health manager, one patient and citizen representative) to consider the case. The IRP encourages locally acceptable solutions. Its advice takes account of public and patient involvement and the rigour of local consultation. As a non-departmental public body, the IRP offers advice only: final decisions rest with the Secretary of State.
www.irpanel.org.uk

Vital statistics: beds in the NHS 2004/05

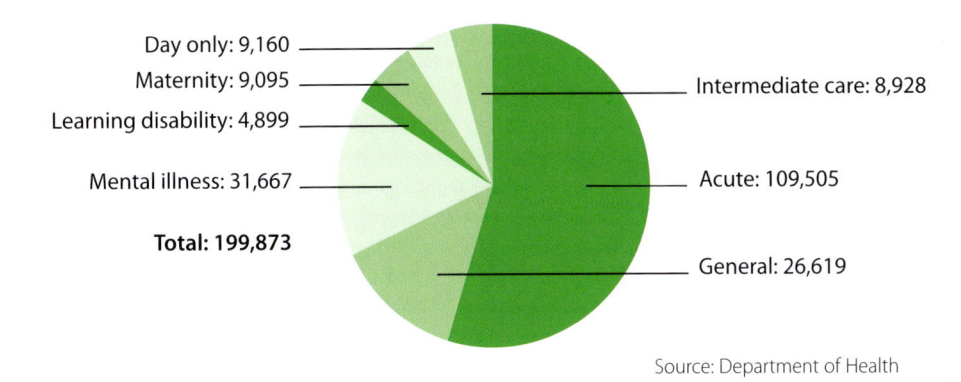

Day only: 9,160
Maternity: 9,095
Learning disability: 4,899
Mental illness: 31,667
Total: 199,873
Intermediate care: 8,928
Acute: 109,505
General: 26,619

Source: Department of Health

A treatment centre's essential features include:
- delivering a high volume of routine treatments and/or diagnostics
- streamlined services using defined pathways
- planned and booked services, with emphasis on patient choice and convenience.

Treatment centres are being developed on two models. Some are run by the NHS, others by the independent sector or overseas providers (see page 29) under contract to the NHS. They may be:
- virtual treatment centres – defined services within an existing hospital, using care pathways to ensure efficiency and enhance the patient's experience
- stand-alone new-build treatment centres – purposely designed for maximum efficiency and to ensure the best patient flows
- refurbished sites – possibly using surplus estate to give quick access to suitable buildings.

The type of work they do falls into three categories:
- short-stay inpatient work, often in a single specialty such as orthopaedics or ophthalmology
- day-case or outpatient work, sometimes referred to as 'surgi-centres'
- community-based diagnostic work, such as endoscopy and ultrasound, and minor surgical procedures such as excision of cysts and lesions, and vasectomies.

> **Key organisation: NHS Elect**

NHS Elect is a confederation of NHS elective care providers. It aims to help improve clinical and operational efficiency by adoption of best international practice, models of public sector marketing and streamlined patient pathways. NHS Elect has access to international expertise in ambulatory care and to overseas doctors who can work in elective care centres. Many of its members have NHS treatment centres, and it supports them in marketing their services to PCTs, GPs and patients. Although it began as a network of four treatment centres pioneering new ways of working, it now supports any NHS organisation providing elective care, and in addition offers a programme to PCTs. www.nhselect.org.uk

Centres may serve patients from a limited catchment area or accept those waiting a long time from anywhere. They may care for patients within a single specialty or a range of specialties. Since 2002, 46 NHS-run treatment centres have opened. More than 30 ISTC sites are fully operational.

Although treatment centres enable the NHS to treat patients more quickly than before, there are concerns that they could cause problems for some hospitals by removing large amounts of their work, so threatening the viability of some of their services. The location and specialty of treatment centres must therefore be decided carefully.

Further information
Treatment centres: delivering faster, quality care and choice for NHS patients, DH, January 2005.

Ambulance services

Emergency care is undergoing major changes, driven by a ten-year strategy, Reforming Emergency Care, launched in 2001.

Ambulance services have changed significantly in the past decade, with big improvements in response times for 999 calls, in training and quality of care, vehicle standards, equipment and technology. But as demand for ambulances is rising by an extra 250,000 responses a year, the Government has set a new

Where care is delivered

strategic direction. The intention is to transform ambulance services from focusing mainly on resuscitation, trauma and acute care to providing more diagnosis, treatment and care in people's homes, helping avoid unnecessary A&E admissions. In 2006, many of the 32 ambulance trusts merged to create 11 new organisations.

Ambulance trust areas

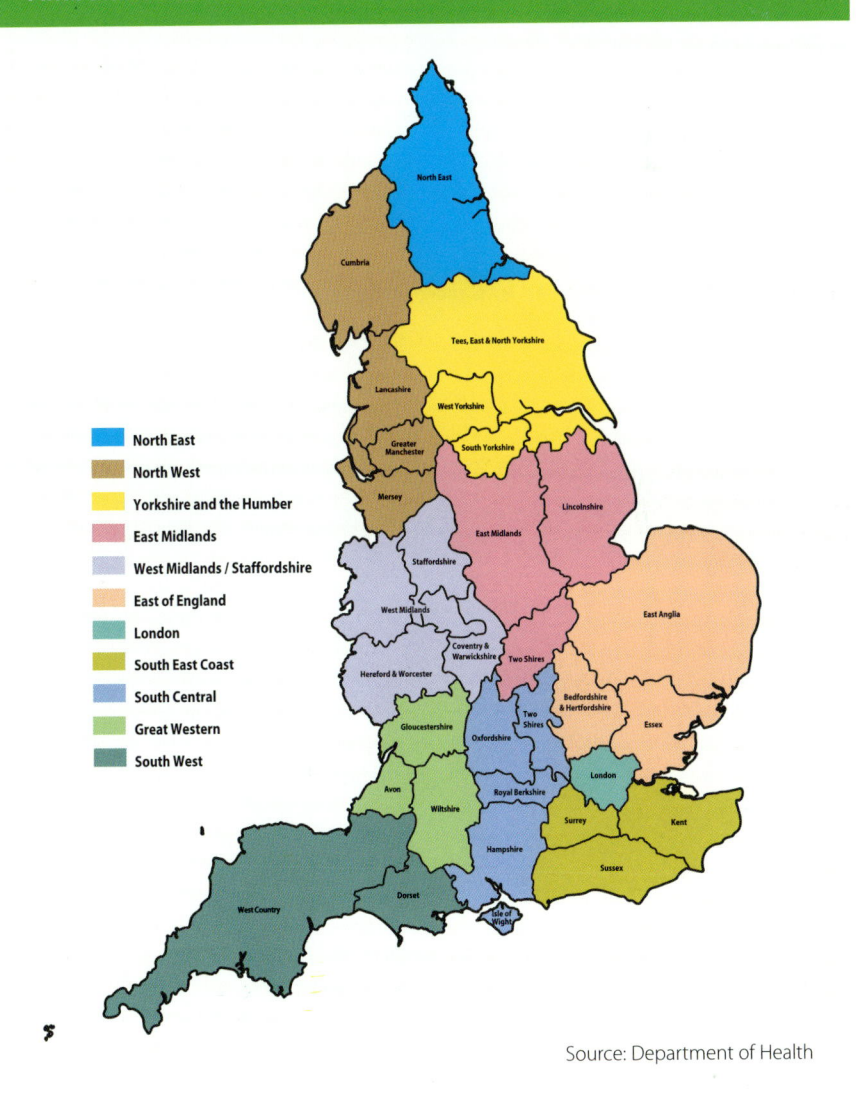

- North East
- North West
- Yorkshire and the Humber
- East Midlands
- West Midlands / Staffordshire
- East of England
- London
- South East Coast
- South Central
- Great Western
- South West

Source: Department of Health

57

NHS ambulances in England made 6 million emergency responses in 2005/06, a 6 per cent increase on the previous year and more than double the number in 1992/93.

Ambulance services respond to 999 calls, doctors' urgent admission requests, high-dependency and inter-hospital transfers, referrals from NHS Direct and major incidents. Key standards for ambulance services include:
- from 2008, responding to all category A (life threatening) calls within eight minutes or less of the call being connected to the control room
- responding to non-life threatening (Category B) calls within 14 minutes in urban areas or 19 minutes in rural areas
- ensuring GP urgent calls arrive at hospital within 15 minutes of the time stipulated by the GP
- thrombolysis (clot-busting drugs) to be delivered within 60 minutes of the call for help.

In many areas ambulance trusts also provide transport to get patients to hospital for non-emergency treatment.

Since 2004, local NHS organisations have discretion over whether their ambulance service should automatically respond to category C calls: for these non-urgent conditions, callers may be referred to another NHS provider or treated at home.

Crews now use satellite navigation systems, and emergency ambulances are equipped with technology such as ECG machines and telemetry, which lets crews send information about a patient's condition directly to the receiving hospital.

The new role of emergency care practitioner has cut across traditional professional boundaries. ECPs respond to 999 calls to provide patients with timely care that may avert a transfer to an A&E department and reduce demand on ambulances. They also support GPs in out-of-hours services by carrying out home visits.

Further information
NHS ambulance services... more than just patient transport, NHS Confederation, July 2006.
Taking healthcare to the patient: transforming NHS ambulance services, DH, June 2005.
Right skill, right time, right place: the ECP report, NHS Modernisation Agency, October 2004.

Mental health

One in four people seek help for a mental health problem at some point in their lives. Mental health is one of the Government's core national priorities (see page 75), with new services and staff being introduced as a result of the NHS Plan.

Organising mental health services

Mental health services are provided as part of primary and secondary care, with responsibility split between the NHS, social services and the independent and voluntary sectors. However, PCTs are responsible for commissioning all mental health services. There are 39 specialist mental health trusts that provide acute inpatient care, community and rehabilitation services, residential care centres, day hospitals and drop-in centres. Some PCTs also provide mental health services: their future role in doing so will evolve as *Commissioning a patient-led NHS* and *Our health, our care, our say* are implemented. About 80,000 staff work in statutory mental health services.

Primary and community services

Of people who receive help for mental health problems, 90 per cent are dealt with in primary care. In a typical PCT of 330,000 people, about 40,000 will suffer from depression, anxiety or other so-called mental disorders. Another 800 will suffer from a psychotic illness such as schizophrenia. Of GP consultations, 30 per cent have a significant mental health component.

Nevertheless, 80 per cent of NHS spending on mental health is devoted to inpatient services. Less than half of GPs have postgraduate training in psychiatry and only 2 per cent of practice nurses have mental health training, although about half of GP surgeries provide counselling. The GMS contract gives GPs an incentive to provide care for the physical health of people with severe mental illness. GPs usually refer patients they cannot help directly to the local community mental health team (CMHT) or to a psychiatric outpatient clinic.

CMHTs – sometimes known as primary care liaison teams – are the main source of specialist support for those suffering severe and enduring mental health problems. They assess and monitor mental health needs using two specialist systems – the care programme approach (currently being reviewed) or care management. These require that everyone seen by specialist mental health services should have their need for treatment assessed, a care plan drawn up and a named mental health worker to co-ordinate their care, including a regular review of their needs. They aim to help provide continuity of care across different services, promote multi-professional and inter-agency working, and ensure appropriate care for people diagnosed with serious mental illness on discharge from hospital.

CMHT members include community psychiatric nurses, social workers, psychologists, occupational therapists, doctors and support workers. Patients will regularly meet the psychiatrist from their mental health team at a psychiatric outpatient clinic for review of their treatment.

Providing mental health services in the community has prompted new approaches to care to avoid hospital admission, such as:
- early intervention teams, which aim to treat psychotic illness as quickly and effectively as possible, especially during the critical period after its onset
- assertive outreach teams to provide intensive support for severely mentally ill people who are difficult to engage in more traditional services
- home treatment and crisis resolution to provide flexible acute care in patients' own homes, with a 24-hour service to help with crises.

Further information
Reviewing the care programme approach 2006: a consultation document, CSIP and DH, November 2006.
Leading edge 17: Adult mental health services in primary care, NHS Confederation, November 2005.

Hospital services
Psychiatric hospital services have been progressively scaled down over the past 30 years, as many services once provided in hospitals are now provided in the community. However, numbers of patients detained under the Mental Health Act have been rising, intensifying pressure on beds and stress on staff. One result of fewer beds and rising demand has been a significant increase in pressure on hospital services, with psychiatric beds experiencing high occupancy rates – more than 100 per cent in about half of wards. Acute inpatient services deal mainly with patients suffering severe mental illness.

Child and adolescent mental health services
Child and adolescent mental health services (CAMHS) cater for young people and children with all types of mental disorder, including hyperkinetic disorders. Services are arranged into four tiers, which should be closely linked:

- tier 1 includes services contributing to mental healthcare of children and young people, but whose primary function is not mental healthcare (for example, schools and GPs)
- tier 2 includes mental health professionals assessing and treating those who do not respond at tier 1
- tier 3 includes teams of mental health professionals providing multi-disciplinary interventions for more complex problems
- tier 4 includes the most severe and complex problems that cannot be dealt with at tier 3, including inpatient and specialist services such as eating disorders.

All areas were required to have 'comprehensive CAMHS' by the end of 2006. This includes out-of-hours emergency cover as well as adequate provision for all young people, up to age 18, with mental health problems.

Further information
Promoting the mental health and psychological well-being of children and young people: report on the implementation of standard 9 of the national service framework for children, young people and maternity services, DH, November 2006.

Forensic services

Forensic mental health services deal with mentally ill people who may need a degree of physical security and have shown challenging behaviour beyond the scope of general psychiatric services. Some may be mentally disordered offenders.

Services fall into three categories:
- low-security services tend to be based near general psychiatric wards in NHS hospitals
- medium-secure services often operate regionally and usually consist of locked wards with a greater number and a wider range of staff
- high-security services are provided by the three special hospitals (Ashworth, Broadmoor and Rampton), which have much greater levels of security and care for people who pose an immediate and serious risk to others.

In addition, new services are developing to meet the needs of mentally disordered offenders in the community.

Modernising services

The National Service Framework for mental health, published in 1999, sets out a ten-year programme to introduce new standards of care that people will be entitled to expect in every part of the country. It emphasises:
- mental health promotion – to ensure health and social services promote mental health and reduce discrimination and social exclusion associated with mental illness
- primary care and access to services – to deliver better primary mental healthcare and ensure consistent help for people with mental health needs, including primary care services for those with severe mental illness
- effective services for people with severe mental illness – to ensure each person receives the services they need, that crises are anticipated or prevented, that help is prompt and effective if a crisis does occur, and access timely to an appropriate and safe mental health place or hospital bed, as close to home as possible
- caring about carers – to ensure health and social services assess carers' needs and provide care to meet their needs
- preventing suicide – to ensure that health and social services play their full part in reducing the suicide rate by at least one-fifth by 2010.

In a five-year assessment of progress, the national director for mental health indicated a need to focus on whole-community mental health.

The DH has now set out a national framework within which patients will have more choice over mental health services. It promises service users the power to choose their own path through services as well as to exercise their preferences over how, when, where and what treatments they receive.

Further information
Our choices in mental health, CSIP and NIMHE, November 2006.
The 2005/06 national survey of investment in mental health services, DH, May 2006.
National service framework for mental health: modern standards and service models, DH, September 1999.
The National Service Framework for mental health – five years on, NHS Confederation, March 2005.
Choices in Mental Health website **www.mhchoice.csip.org.uk**

Delivering race equality in mental healthcare

This initiative was launched in 2005 and outlines a five-year action plan for achieving equality and tackling discrimination in mental health services in England and for all people of black and minority ethnic (BME) status. Delivering race equality (DRE) is part of a wider programme of action to develop greater equality in health and social care. The programme is based on three building blocks:
- providing more appropriate and responsive services and improving clinical services for specific groups, such as older people, asylum seekers, refugees and children
- engaging communities in planning services, supported by 500 new community development workers
- improving ethnicity monitoring, dissemination of information and knowledge about effective services, including a regular census of mental health patients.

The vision for DRE is that by 2010 there will be a service characterised by 'less fear' among BME communities and service users; increased satisfaction with services; a reduced rate of admission of people from BME communities to psychiatric inpatient units; a reduction in the disproportionate rates of compulsory detention of BME service users in inpatient units and a more balanced range of culturally appropriate and effective therapies.

Focused implementation sites have been established to help identify and spread best practice. The evaluation of these sites in 2008 will inform national implementation. A BME mental health programme board, directly accountable to ministers, is overseeing this action plan and the wider BME mental health programme.

Further information
Briefing 138: Commissioning race equality in mental health care, NHS Confederation, October 2006.

Revising mental health law

The Government is in the process of amending the Mental Health Act 1983. The Mental Health Bill 2006 contains these changes:
- supervised treatment in the community to ensure that patients who have been detained and treated in hospital comply with treatment, so helping to prevent relapse and readmission to hospital
- broadening the range of professionals who can take on key roles in the Mental Health Act

- order-making powers with regard to the Mental Health Review Tribunal – precise changes are still under consultation
- enabling patients to apply to the county court to appoint an acting nearest relative where they have reasonable objections to the person who would otherwise have that role
- powers to reduce the time for referral to the Mental Health Review Tribunal for all civil patients who do not apply for a tribunal
- a new, simplified single definition of mental disorder so that no one is denied treatment because they do not fall within the existing legal categories of mental disorder – for example, people with personality disorders
- a new criterion for compulsion, that appropriate treatment must be available before a patient can be detained; this replaces the 'treatability' test
- ending finite restriction orders, so that restrictions will remain in force for as long as the offender's mental disorder poses a risk of harm to others
- by amending the Mental Capacity Act 2005, introduction of the 'Bournewood safeguards' for people who lack capacity to make decisions for themselves, and are deprived of their liberty in care homes or hospital, but do not receive mental health legislation safeguards.

Involving patients and the public

Involving patients and the public in health services can be interpreted in different ways.
- Individual patients may be involved together with health professionals in making decisions about their own care.
- Users of a particular service may be involved as a group in advising how it might be improved.
- Members of the public may be involved in making strategic decisions about how or where services are to be provided.

The NHS Plan aimed to ensure patients and the public have a real say in how services are planned and developed. The Health and Social Care Act 2001 places a duty on health authorities, primary care trusts and NHS trusts to 'involve and consult' patients and the public. They were already required by law to consult on substantial variations and developments to services; under the Act, they must arrange to involve and consult patients and the public in:
- planning services they are responsible for

- developing and considering proposals for changes in the way those services are provided
- decisions to be made that affect how those services operate.

In *Health reform in England: update and commissioning framework* (see page XX), the Government announced that the Act's requirements for consulting patients and public would be made more explicit.

This means discussing with patients and the public their ideas, the organisation's plans, patients' experiences, why services need to change, what people want from services and how to make best use of resources. Boards must consider patient and public involvement issues on their agendas, include among their membership an individual to champion these issues and designate a staff member responsible for the activity. They must commit resources to patient and public involvement, and ensure all staff are trained in it. In 2006 the white paper, *Our health, our care, our say*, called for 'a more rigorous fulfilment of existing duties to involve and consult the public in how services are provided'.

The NHS Plan requires every trust to obtain feedback from patients about their experiences of care. In addition, the Healthcare Commission (see page 82) is responsible for a programme of national patient surveys (see pages 95). Information from patient surveys is used in assessing trusts' performance. Sweeping reforms to the structure of patient and public involvement created new

Key organisation: NHS Centre for Involvement

Founded in 2006, this national centre is intended to help NHS staff and organisations involve patients and public in their local health services. It hopes to become 'a one-stop shop for information and advice on PPI', including an advice and enquiry service able to offer evidence on what works and models of good practice. The centre is run by a consortium comprising Warwick University, the Centre for Public Scrutiny and the Long-term Medical Conditions Alliance. It works closely with the NHS Institute for Innovation and Improvement, which is responsible for managing its performance.
www.nhscentreforinvolvement.nhs.uk

bodies, outlined below, to replace the community health councils that had existed since 1974. In addition, local authority overview and scrutiny committees (see page 146) are intended to ensure elected councillors have a say in the NHS in their area, while the public can become members of foundation trusts and elect representatives to the board of governors (see page 37).

Further information
Patient and public involvement in health: the evidence for policy implementation, DH, May 2004.

Patient advice and liaison services

Every NHS trust and primary care trust should have a patient advice and liaison service (PALS) providing on-the-spot help and information about health services. PALS aim to:
- resolve concerns before they become major problems
- provide information to patients, carers and their families about local health services and put people in contact with local support groups
- tell people about the complaints procedure and independent complaints advocacy support
- act as an early-warning system by monitoring trends, highlighting gaps in service and making reports for action to trust managers.

The National PALS Development Group comprises representatives of PALS staff from each SHA area, and shares learning and best practice. The National PALS office is located in Macclesfield.

Further information
National evaluation of PALS: briefing for chief executives, University of the West of England and DH, September 2006.
PALS Online **www.pals.nhs.uk**

Local involvement networks (LINks)

LINks will become the successor bodies to patient and public involvement forums (PPIFs), but will differ from them in several ways. They will cover a geographical area rather than relate to a specific organisation, and will cover both health and social care. It is intended they will involve many more people and work more closely with the voluntary sector than PPIFs. LINks will also be given the power to inspect premises: it is proposed that each LINk will have a team of specialists trained for this.

Key texts

Kennedy Report
The inquiry into the deaths of child heart patients at Bristol Royal Infirmary from 1984 to 1995 was chaired by Professor Sir Ian Kennedy and made many important recommendations for change in the NHS, not least that there should be representation of patient interests on the inside of the NHS and at every level. It was published in 2001.
www.bristol-inquiry.org.uk

The Expert Patient
This DH policy document published in 2001 defined a new relationship between patient and professional, in which 'the era of the patient as the passive recipient of healthcare is changing and being replaced by a new emphasis on the relationship between the NHS and the people whom it serves'. In 2006 the DH announced that it intended to expand its Expert Patients programme from 12,000 course places a year to over 100,000 by 2012, and has created a community interest company for that purpose.
www.expertpatients.nhs.uk

Before the advent of PPIFs, community health councils acted as patient and public representatives in England until they were abolished in 2003. They continue in Wales with new powers. NHSScotland has replaced its local health councils with a single Scottish Health Council that has local offices in each board area, while Northern Ireland plans a single Patient and Client Council to replace its four health and social service councils.

Further information
A stronger local voice: a framework for creating a stronger local voice in the development of health and social care services – a document for information and comment, DH, July 2006.
Government response to 'A stronger local voice', DH, December 2006.

National director for patients and the public
The Department of Health created a post of national director for patients and the public in 2003. The director's role is to:

- champion the voice of patients, carers and the public throughout the NHS and in the DH
- support staff to work in partnership with patients and carers, and be responsive to their needs
- act as a national spokesperson in promoting and explaining patient-focused policy.

The director reports to the chief nursing officer, who has lead responsibility for patient and public involvement.

Spotlight on policy: patient choice

The Government wants the NHS to offer more convenient, 'personalised care' that takes account of patients' preferences concerning where and when they are treated. Since January 2006, patients have had the right to be offered a choice of at least four locations, including one in the private sector, when they need to be referred by their GP for further treatment. In addition to local options commissioned by their PCT, patients may now choose from a 'national menu' of services offered by the 'extended choice network' of providers made up of NHS foundation trusts, the first wave of ISTCs and other nationally appointed independent providers. By mid-2007, over 200 hospitals should be in the scheme, and by 2008 patients will be able to choose from any hospital or provider that meets NHS standards and costs.

Booklets about local hospitals are available to help patients make their choice. These include information on waiting times, MRSA rates, access and cancelled operations. Patients may choose a hospital and an appointment time during the consultation with their GP, or book later by phone or internet. By the end of 2006, more than 85 per cent of GP practices were making referrals through Choose and Book (see page 137).

A DH survey in July 2006 found 32 per cent of patients were aware beforehand they had a choice of hospitals for their first appointment, while 75 per cent offered choice were satisfied with the process.

The strategy paper, *Building on the best*, outlined other aspects of patient choice that the Government wants to see, some of which has now been implemented.

Spotlight on policy: patient choice continued

It included:
- new ways to access primary care, including nurse-led clinics and polyclinics offering a wide range of GP and specialist services. Diagnostic tests formerly carried out only in hospital will be available here, performed by GPs, nurses and others with specialist interests
- commuters able to register with a GP near their work, instead of at home
- patients able to get repeat prescriptions for medicines from a pharmacist of their choice for up to a year, without having to go back to their GP. By 2007, new IT arrangements will enable patients to pick up repeat medicines from any pharmacy in England. The range of over-the-counter medicines available without prescription will be expanded, making it easier for patients to manage their own conditions
- local services promoting direct access to midwives
- patients able to enter preferences on to their own electronic care record.

Giving patients greater choice is a key priority for the NHS. It holds out the prospect of a more responsive service tailored around the individual, with patients as genuine partners in decisions about their care. However, it requires explicit statements about options available to patients, which will involve debate about priorities for investment and the limits to choice. Without a wider programme of culture change, increased choice may be insufficient to improve the responsiveness of the system. To ensure equity, policies will need to be targeted at those unable to exercise choice: case managers and advisers to help patients navigate the system will be important in this.

Further information
Choice matters: increasing choice improves patients' experiences – patients, GPs and practice managers talk about their experiences of choice and Choose and Book, DH, May 2006.
Choice at referral: guidance framework for 2006/7, DH, April 2006.
'Choose & Book' – patient's choice of hospital and booked appointment, DH, August 2004.
Building on the best; choice, equity and responsiveness in the NHS, DH, December 2003.

3

NHS strategy: putting policy in context

A framework for reform

The NHS in England has been fundamentally redefined since 1997, moving from a comprehensive system of state funding and public provision to a mixed economy of public, private and voluntary providers – though still state-funded. All current policy initiatives need to be set in this context, where provision is becoming increasingly pluralistic and diverse.

The Government argues in the NHS operating framework for 2007/08 that its reforms are not a response to 'some centrally driven agenda' but to rising expectations, an ageing population, changes in medical technology and the need to tackle variations in quality, safety, access and value for money. Its strategy is to address these challenges through:
- more choice for patients, backed by stronger commissioning
- more diverse providers, with greater freedom to innovate and more competition on quality
- financial incentives to improve care and promote sound financial management and best value
- national standards and regulation to guarantee quality, safety and equity
- a sustained focus on information management and technology.

The overall aim is a 'patient-led' NHS that is 'self-improving' – where innovation and improvement are 'in-built'. The reforms are designed to achieve 'the right balance of incentives, patient choice, plurality and transparency in the system' to bring this about, the Government says.

Nevertheless, risks lie ahead: of improvements in efficiency at the expense of quality; the fragmentation of care requiring complex co-ordination; further marginalisation of socially excluded groups and massive changes in local services. No one has a complete understanding of the possible effects of the current policy mix sufficient to guarantee that potentially dysfunctional consequences will not occur.

Further information
The NHS in England: the operating framework for 2007/08, DH, December 2006.
Briefing 129: Health reform – the agenda for 2006, NHS Confederation, March 2006.
Health reform in England: update and next steps, DH, December 2005.

The planning framework

Public service agreement

Every two years the Treasury conducts a spending review of all Government departments, which spans three years (the third year being carried over to become the first year of the following plan). The Chancellor then announces each department's settlement, and each department draws up a public service agreement (PSA) with the Treasury, setting out what it is expected to provide with its new resources over the three-year period. PSAs are the main way in which the Government tries to ensure that increased resources secure public service reform and improved performance.

The aim of the Department of Health's current PSA, published after the 2004 spending review, is to 'transform the health and social care system so that it produces faster, fairer services that deliver better health and tackle health inequalities'. It sets four objectives, to:
- improve the health of the population
- improve health outcomes for people with long-term conditions
- improve access to services
- improve the patient and user experience.

This latest PSA reconfigured the targets set in previous ones, with longer-term targets being carried forward, those already met converted into established standards and new targets being created to reflect evolving priorities.

During 2007 the Government intends to conduct its second comprehensive spending review (the first was in 1998), which 'will represent a long-term and fundamental review' of public expenditure. It will cover departmental allocations for 2008/09, 2009/10 and 2010/11.

In addition, the DH's priorities for 2006/07 are contained in its business plan. These are:
- to lead sustained improvements in public health and well-being, especially for disadvantaged and vulnerable people
- to enhance the quality and safety of health and social care services, providing faster access and better patient and user choice and control
- to improve patients' and users' experience of care, including those with long-term conditions
- to improve the capacity, capability and efficiency of the health and social care system
- to ensure that systems reform, service modernisation, IT investment and new staff contracts improve quality and value for money
- to improve the service provided to – and on behalf of – the public, nationally and internationally
- to develop departmental capability and efficiency.

Further information
Department of Health business plan 2006–07, DH, December 2006.
Department of Health autumn performance report, CM6985, HMSO, December 2006.
2004 Spending Review: public service agreements 2005–2008, HM Treasury, July 2004.
2007 Comprehensive Spending Review **http://csr07.treasury.gov.uk/**

Future objectives for the NHS

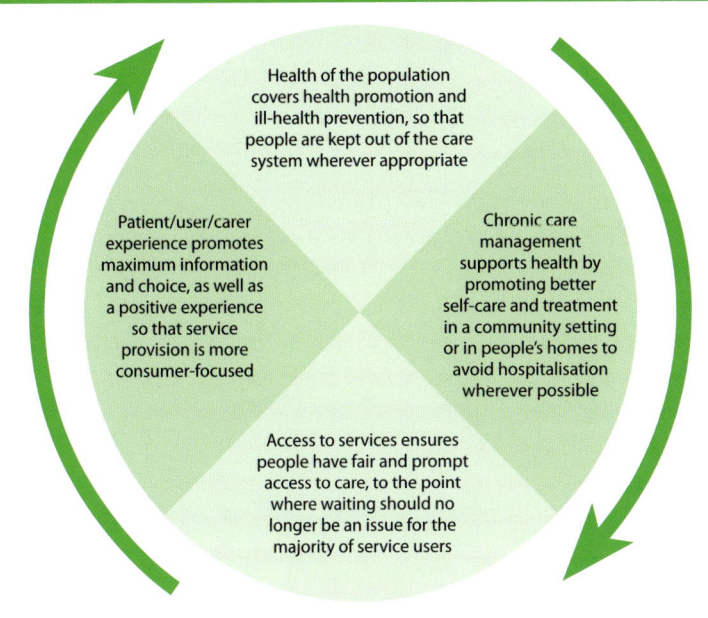

Health of the population covers health promotion and ill-health prevention, so that people are kept out of the care system wherever appropriate

Patient/user/carer experience promotes maximum information and choice, as well as a positive experience so that service provision is more consumer-focused

Chronic care management supports health by promoting better self-care and treatment in a community setting or in people's homes to avoid hospitalisation wherever possible

Access to services ensures people have fair and prompt access to care, to the point where waiting should no longer be an issue for the majority of service users

Source: *NHS Improvement Plan,* Department of Health 2004

Priorities and planning framework

The DH translates PSA objectives into a priorities and planning framework for the NHS and social services covering three years, so that organisations can look in depth at their services, plan change confidently and implement improvements year on year. Each organisation needs to follow six steps:
- identifying national and local priorities and key targets
- agreeing capacity
- deciding each health and social care organisation's specific responsibilities
- creating robust plans and involving staff and the public in them
- setting up sound arrangements to monitor progress
- improving communication and accountability.

Responsibilities are divided between health and social services. The NHS leads on developing plans for improving access, improving services for cancer, coronary heart disease, improving the patient experience, alleviating health inequalities and drug misuse. Local government directors of children's services lead on improving life chances for children. The NHS and social services lead jointly on mental health and services for older people. Strategic health authorities oversee the planning process and outcome where the NHS is leading. Primary care trusts and councils should agree arrangements where the lead is joint.

Local delivery plans (LDPs)

NHS planning is intended to take place from the bottom up, although within a fairly prescriptive national framework. In 2005 the DH reduced the number of national targets from 62 to 20 to give PCTs more 'headroom' to set local ones, which will not be monitored by the DH but the Healthcare Commission. However, for the 2008 planning round, the DH and SHAs will only agree PCTs' LDPs if they demonstrate a clear strategy for developing preventive services – including ambitious goals for shifting resources – as set out in the white paper, *Our health, our care, our say*.

PCTs develop plans with the help of clinicians as well as patients and the public. SHAs bring together PCT plans to make a comprehensive LDP, which should cover acute trusts.

The LDP identifies expected progress for each priority area over the three-year planning period, specifying quarterly or annual milestones or even – for a few critical features – planned progress on a month-by-month basis. The LDP is supported by a financial strategy and plan showing how resources are to be deployed and value for money achieved. Although an LDP covers a whole SHA area, it is based on PCT-level plans and must take account of practice-based commissioning. It is intended to be a 'live' document that is amended on an ongoing basis if corrective action has to be taken or new initiatives are begun.

The SHA-level LDPs form the basis of the management relationship between the NHS and the DH. The LDPs show how each area plans to achieve the national targets and key capacity increases. In line with the Government's spending review cycle, plans are completely updated every two years, with year three of the existing plan becoming year one of the new plan.

Key issues for 2007/08

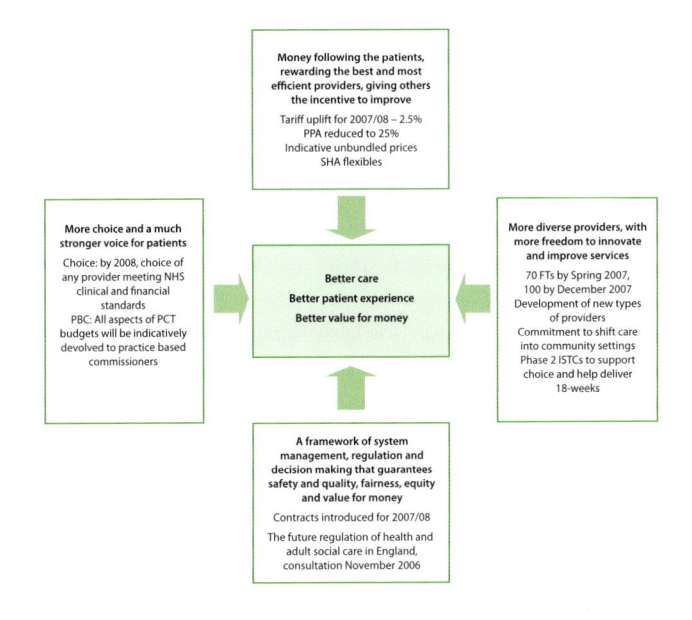

Money following the patients, rewarding the best and most efficient providers, giving others the incentive to improve
Tariff uplift for 2007/08 – 2.5%
PPA reduced to 25%
Indicative unbundled prices
SHA flexibles

More choice and a much stronger voice for patients
Choice: by 2008, choice of any provider meeting NHS clinical and financial standards
PBC: All aspects of PCT budgets will be indicatively devolved to practice based commissioners

Better care
Better patient experience
Better value for money

More diverse providers, with more freedom to innovate and improve services
70 FTs by Spring 2007,
100 by December 2007
Development of new types of providers
Commitment to shift care into community settings
Phase 2 ISTCs to support choice and help deliver 18-weeks

A framework of system management, regulation and decision making that guarantees safety and quality, fairness, equity and value for money
Contracts introduced for 2007/08
The future regulation of health and adult social care in England, consultation November 2006

Source: The NHS in England: the operating framework for 2007/08, Department of Health 2006

Priorities 2005–08

National priorities for the NHS and social services' for the three financial years 2005/06 to 2007/08, based on the DH's PSA, are:
- *improve the health of the population:* increasing life expectancy at birth in England to 78.6 years for men and to 82.5 years for women by 2010
- *support people with long-term conditions:* by offering a personalised care plan for vulnerable people most at risk and reducing emergency bed-days by 5 per cent by 2008
- *access to services:* ensuring that by 2008 no one waits more than 18 weeks from GP referral to hospital treatment; increasing problem drug-users' participation in drug treatment programmes by 100 per cent by 2008
- *patient/user experience:* ensuring that individuals are fully involved in decisions about their care, including choice of provider; supporting vulnerable older people to live in their own homes; reducing MRSA levels and other healthcare-associated infections.

Within each priority area are several key targets, relevant to primary care as well as hospital services and achievable only with close co-operation between health and social services. In addition, local communities have their own priorities, as do local authorities.

Commitments from the 2003–06 planning round extend into the new planning round. PCTs and partner organisations are expected to deliver these commitments by their target dates and maintain performance after that. The Healthcare Commission monitors these achievements.

Issues for particular attention in 2006/07 were:
- *health inequalities:* with an initial focus on smoking cessation
- *shorter waits for cancer services:* reducing the maximum waiting time from urgent referral to treatment to 62 days, and achieving a maximum waiting time of 31 days from diagnosis to treatment for all cancers
- *18-week maximum wait:* from GP referral to hospital treatment by 2008
- *MRSA:* achieving a fall in MRSA levels as set out in local delivery plans
- *patient choice and booking:* every hospital appointment to be booked for the patient's convenience by implementing Choose and Book
- *sexual health and access to genito-urinary medicine clinics:* ensuring that by 2008 everyone referred to a GUM clinic should have an appointment within 48 hours.

In addition, the NHS's operating framework in England stipulates as 'development priorities' in 2007/08:
- further progress towards the 18-week maximum wait from GP referral to treatment: by March 2008, 85 per cent of patients admitted for hospital treatment and 90 per cent of patients not needing admission should be treated within 18 weeks
- continued reduction in hospital-acquired infections, including a new drive on *Clostridium difficile,* with targets agreed locally
- achieving financial health and delivering a net surplus of £250 million across the NHS by the end of 2007/08
- reducing health inequalities and promoting health and well-being, with targets agreed locally.

Further information
The NHS in England: the operating framework for 2007/08, DH, December 2006.
National standards, local action: health and social care standards and planning framework 2005/06–2007/08, DH, July 2004.
Department of Health annual performance report 2005, DH, December 2005.
The NHS in England: the operating framework for 2006/7, DH, January 2006.

Key strategies: key texts, 1997–2006

The new NHS – modern, dependable
The Labour Government's first health white paper after coming to power, published in December 1997. It announced the setting up of primary care groups (forerunners of PCTs), NICE, the Commission for Health Improvement (forerunner of the Healthcare Commission) and NHS Direct, describing reforms that would be 'a new model for a new century'.

The NHS Plan
The NHS Plan is the foundation of the Government's reforms for modernising the health service, and links change explicitly to extra investment announced in the March 2000 Budget. Published in July 2000 and intended as an ambitious ten-year programme, the Plan set out to tackle 'systematic problems, which date from 1948 when the NHS was formed'.

Shifting the balance of power within the NHS
Two documents – *Securing delivery* (July 2001) and *The next steps* (January 2002) – outline the rationale behind devolving power from Whitehall to frontline NHS organisations, in particular PCTs. They announced that SHAs were to replace the existing 95 health authorities and that the DH would have a reduced role in directly managing the NHS.

Key strategies: key texts, 1997–2006 continued

Delivering the NHS Plan: next steps on investment, next steps on reform
This document, published in April 2002, introduced plans to reform the NHS's financial flows through payment by results, brought new emphasis to patient choice and underlined commitment to promoting diversity in supply of healthcare through joint ventures with the private sector.

The NHS Improvement Plan: putting people at the heart of public services
Published in June 2004, this 'supports the ongoing commitment to a ten-year process of reform first set out in the NHS Plan' but adds some new priorities to be achieved by 2008: giving patients more information and extending patient choice through 'personalised care', improving support for people with long-term conditions and stronger emphasis on disease prevention.

Creating a patient-led NHS: delivering the NHS Improvement Plan
In this document, published in March 2005, the Government revealed it wanted 'some radically different types of provision' that would 'involve freeing up the entrepreneurialism within primary care and developing new types of provider organisations'.

Our health, our care, our say
Published in January 2006 (see page 40), this sets out the Government's vision for more effective health and social care services outside hospitals.

Health reform in England: update and commissioning framework
In July 2006, six years after the NHS Plan was published, this document reported on progress and set out commissioning arrangements for hospital services covered by choice and payment by results.

4

NHS quality: improving healthcare

Organisations' responsibility for quality

This Government's first health policy white paper, *The new NHS: modern, dependable*, published in 1997, promised that the service 'will have quality at its heart'. NHS organisations now have a statutory duty to ensure the quality of their services, just as they have always had to keep their organisations financially solvent. NHS trust chief executives are accountable for clinical standards, and each trust has a designated senior clinician who must make sure clinical governance systems are functioning properly. Primary care trusts have to nominate a senior health professional, usually a GP, to lead on clinical standards and professional development. In essence, NHS organisations must:
- develop an open and participative culture
- demonstrate a commitment to quality
- work routinely with patients, users, carers and the public
- encourage an ethos of multidisciplinary team-working at all levels
- reduce unjustifiable variations in quality of care
- share good practice
- detect and deal with poor performance and adverse events.

The Government's aim is to provide clear, national standards for services supported by consistent evidence-based guidance to raise quality, and to put in place a robust system of inspection.

Clinical governance

Clinical governance is an explicit framework for making all NHS staff accountable for quality improvement and safeguarding standards, ensuring that quality remains a priority. The chief medical officer's definition of clinical governance is:

> a system through which NHS organisations are accountable for continuously improving the quality of their services and safeguarding high standards of care, by creating an environment in which clinical excellence will flourish.

Clinical governance seeks to transform the culture, ways of working and systems of every health organisation so that patient safety, quality assurance and improvement are an integral part of their everyday work. Its main features are a coherent approach to quality improvement, clear lines of accountability for clinical quality systems and effective processes for identifying and managing risk and addressing poor performance.

Its essential components are:
- the patient's experience – of access to services, organisation of care, the humanity of care and the environment in which care is delivered
- the organisation's use of information
- consultation and patient involvement
- risk management
- clinical audit
- effectiveness and research
- staffing and staff management
- education, training and continuing professional development
- leadership
- direction and planning, accountability and structures
- partnership with the public
- partnership with the local health economy.

For clinical governance to work properly and quality to flourish, NHS organisations must foster a culture of openness and participation, value education and research, and encourage people to learn from failures. Good practice and new approaches should be shared readily and received willingly.

Key organisation: QQUIP

The Quest for Quality and Improved Performance is a five-year, £2.5 million research initiative organised by the Health Foundation, an independent charitable organisation working to improve healthcare quality across the UK. QQUIP has been set up to help answer three questions about healthcare in England:
- what is the current state of quality and performance?
- what works to improve quality and performance?
- are we getting value for money from what is spent on the NHS?

Its website brings together data to reveal national and international trends on diseases, care quality and the cost-effectiveness of treatments and Government reforms. It is aimed at healthcare policy-makers, researchers, clinicians, managers and patient groups.
www.health.org.uk/qquip

Further information
Improving quality and safety – progress in implementing clinical governance in primary care: lessons for the new primary care trusts, National Audit Office, January 2007. NHS Clinical Governance Support Team www.cgsupport.nhs.uk

Developing integrated governance

NHS boards' decisions must take note not only of clinical governance but of corporate governance, research governance, information governance and financial governance. These strands of governance have developed independently from each other, and do not necessarily align or inter-relate: for example, financial allocations may not always take fully into account the pressures of clinical governance. But, in reality, these domains all complement and impact on one another. Creating different structures to manage and monitor them can lead to duplication and wasted effort, overburdening staff with demands for data.

Some NHS organisations have begun to streamline their governance activities, and several models are emerging – for example, where risk management is a function of the clinical governance committee, or where a single committee embraces controls assurance, clinical governance and risk management. However, integrating the strands of governance is not easy, and much detail remains to be worked out.

Key organisation: the Healthcare Commission

The Healthcare Commission is independent of the Government and reports to Parliament. Its main duties are:
- assessing the management, provision and quality of NHS healthcare, including public health
- reviewing every trust's performance and awarding an annual performance rating
- publishing information about the state of healthcare
- considering complaints about NHS organisations that cannot be resolved locally
- promoting the co-ordination of reviews and assessments carried out by others
- regulating the independent healthcare sector through registration, annual inspection and enforcement
- investigating serious failures in the provision of healthcare.

The Commission co-ordinates the activity of other bodies involved in inspecting healthcare, and has agreed a concordat aimed at reducing the burden of inspection on frontline healthcare staff. This commits each inspectorate to minimising disruption and duplication, ensuring information is shared and encouraging joint inspections. The Commission also operates in Wales.

As part of the Government's drive for a 'balanced regulatory regime' that minimises 'bureaucracy', the Commission will merge with the Commission for Social Care Inspection by 2008, and once legislation is passed it will also take over the functions of the Mental Health Act Commission to create a 'genuinely new regulator'.

Further information
Simplification plan, DH, December 2006.
The future regulation of health and adult social care in England, DH, November 2006.
www.healthcarecommission.org.uk

National service frameworks

National service frameworks (NSFs) are evidence-based programmes setting quality standards and specifying services that should be available for a particular condition or care group across the whole NHS. They are intended to eradicate local variations in standards and services, raise standards generally, promote collaboration between organisations and contribute to improving public health. Each identifies key interventions, puts in place a strategy to support implementation and establishes an agreed timescale.

Each NSF is developed with assistance from an external reference group of health professionals, service users and carers, health service managers, partner agencies and other advocates. The DH supports the groups and manages the overall process.

Usually only one new NSF is released in a year. The programme, begun in 1998, so far covers:
- mental health, September 1999
- coronary heart disease, March 2000
- cancer, September 2000; a new cancer reform strategy is now under development
- older people, March 2001
- diabetes: standards, December 2001; delivery strategy, January 2003
- renal services: part one, January 2004; part two, February 2005
- children, young people and maternity services, September 2004
- long-term conditions, March 2005
- chronic obstructive pulmonary disease, due 2008.

Performance assessment

The current performance framework for the NHS and social care came into effect in April 2005, and replaced the star ratings. The 'annual health check' sets out the level of quality that all organisations providing NHS care – including foundation trusts and those in the private and voluntary sectors – are expected to meet or aspire to. It is administered by the Healthcare Commission. *National standards, local action* set out 24 core standards and 13 developmental standards for NHS organisations. These standards were introduced in 2004 and cover seven 'domains' of activity:
- safety
- care environment and amenities
- clinical and cost-effectiveness
- governance

Key texts

A first class service: quality in the new NHS
Published in June 1998, this provides the blueprint for ensuring quality. Its main themes are the importance of national consistency in implementing evidence-based practice, accountability for local best practice, commitment to a coherent system of quality improvement and assurance, provision for managing poor performance and professional collaboration and teamwork.

An organisation with a memory
Compiled by an expert group led by the chief medical officer and published in June 2000, this recommended a mandatory reporting scheme for adverse healthcare events and near-misses. It set out to encourage a reporting and questioning culture in the NHS to replace blame with a proper understanding of the underlying causes of failures.

Safety first – a report for patients, clinicians and healthcare managers
Commissioned by the chief medical officer and published in December 2006, this updates progress since *An organisation with a memory* and says more remains to be done to ensure patient safety. Its recommendations include a patient safety forum, refocusing the role of the National Patient Safety Agency (see page 88), setting up local patient safety action teams and ensuring national priorities take explicit account of patient safety from 2008.

- patient focus
- accessible and responsive care
- public health.

The DH intends that the core standards serve as 'a platform or "bottom rung" for progress against the developmental ladder'. Performance is also assessed on whether organisations are delivering standards contained in national service frameworks and guidance from the National Institute for Health and Clinical Excellence (see page 87).

The Healthcare Commission examines two areas:
- *getting the basics right* – which includes core standards; national targets; financial position and management; value for money; findings from other regulatory bodies.
- *making and sustaining progress* – including the four national priorities in the DH PSA (see page 71); 'improvement reviews' of patient experiences.

Organisations regulate themselves against the Commission's standards, with local partner bodies and patient forums helping monitor performance. The Commission carries out spot checks and unannounced visits to verify data. Inspections are targeted wherever concerns exist. It also takes account of information from other organisations such as the Commission for Social Care Inspection and the Mental Health Act Commission.

The Healthcare Commission has a statutory duty to produce an annual performance rating for every NHS organisation, and strives to publish information in a way that 'people can understand and use'. The result is a two-part rating based on quality of services and use of resources, including finance, property and staff. Ratings are published on a four-point scale: excellent, good, fair, or weak.

Ratings for each organisation are published every October. In 2005/06, 4 per cent of NHS trusts got the highest rating of 'excellent' for quality of services, 36 per cent were rated 'good', 51 per cent 'fair' and 9 per cent were 'weak'. For use of resources, 3 per cent were 'excellent', 12 per cent 'good', 47 per cent 'fair' and 37 per cent were 'weak'. In the independent acute sector, 6 per cent met all 32 core standards, 33 per cent met at least 29 and 6 per cent failed to meet five or more core standards.

After consultation, the Commission redesigned the health check for 2006/07, increasing its attention to how services are improving while continuing to focus on 'getting the basics right'. It will also assess performance on these specific topics:
- maternity
- diabetes
- substance misuse
- adult acute inpatient mental healthcare
- race equality
- learning disabilities
- complaints handling
- healthcare-acquired infection.

The annual health check in 2006/07

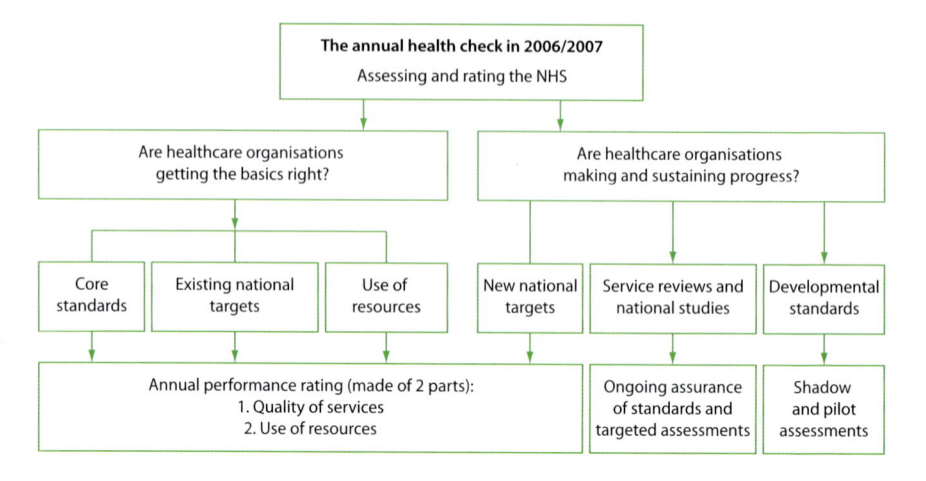

```
                    The annual health check in 2006/2007
                       Assessing and rating the NHS

       ┌─────────────────────────────┐    ┌─────────────────────────────┐
       │ Are healthcare organisations│    │ Are healthcare organisations│
       │   getting the basics right? │    │making and sustaining progress?│
       └─────────────────────────────┘    └─────────────────────────────┘

  ┌────────┬──────────────┬──────────┐    ┌──────────┬──────────────┬──────────────┐
  │ Core   │ Existing     │ Use of   │    │ New      │ Service      │ Developmental│
  │standards│ national    │resources │    │ national │ reviews and  │ standards    │
  │        │ targets      │          │    │ targets  │ national     │              │
  │        │              │          │    │          │ studies      │              │
  └────────┴──────────────┴──────────┘    └──────────┴──────────────┴──────────────┘

  ┌───────────────────────────────────┐    ┌────────────────┬────────────┐
  │ Annual performance rating         │    │ Ongoing        │ Shadow     │
  │ (made of 2 parts):                │    │ assurance of   │ and pilot  │
  │ 1. Quality of services            │    │ standards and  │ assessments│
  │ 2. Use of resources               │    │ targeted       │            │
  │                                   │    │ assessments    │            │
  └───────────────────────────────────┘    └────────────────┴────────────┘
```

Source: Healthcare Commission

Further information
The annual health check in 2006/2007 – assessing and rating the NHS, Healthcare Commission, September 2006.
State of healthcare report 2006, Healthcare Commission, October 2006.
National standards, local action: health and social care standards and planning framework 2005/06–2007/08, DH, July 2004.

Reforming clinical negligence procedures

Although the NHS provides high-quality healthcare for millions of people every year, occasionally patients do not receive the treatment they should, or mistakes are made. About 10 per cent of hospital inpatient admissions may result in some kind of adverse event, while 5 per cent of the population report suffering some injury or other adverse effects of medical care; almost a third of those claim it had a permanent impact on their health. About 18 per cent of patients say they suffered a medication error some time in the previous two years.

Anyone who suffers harm as a result of treatment must receive an apology, a clear explanation of what went wrong, proper treatment and care and, where appropriate, financial compensation. The NHS must ensure it learns from such experiences.

Key organisation: National Institute for Health and Clinical Excellence

Set up in 1999, NICE took over the Health Development Agency's responsibilities in 2005 and now provides national guidance on promoting good health as well as preventing and treating ill health. Its guidance covers three areas:
- technology appraisals – on the use of new and existing medicines and treatments in the NHS in England and Wales.
- clinical guidelines – on the appropriate treatment of specific conditions in the NHS in England and Wales.
- interventional procedures – on whether procedures for diagnosis or treatment are safe enough and work well enough for routine use in England, Wales and Scotland.

In Scotland a special health board, NHS Quality Improvement Scotland, combines many of the roles performed in England by the Healthcare Commission and NICE.

The DH commissions NICE to examine specific topics, which may be suggested by patients, the public, health professionals, the national clinical directors or the National Horizon Scanning Centre (see page 217). Health professionals and the NHS are expected to take NICE guidance fully into account, although it does not override their responsibility to make appropriate decisions based on individual patients' circumstances. NHS organisations in England and Wales must fund medicines and treatments recommended by NICE in technology appraisals. Local government and NHS organisations must take account of NICE public health guidance in working towards the targets in the *Choosing health* white paper (see page 152) and in local area agreements.

NICE's 30-strong citizens' council keeps the organisation informed on what the public thinks about the use of treatments and NHS care. Members are drawn from all age groups, social circumstances, ethnic backgrounds, regions and abilities. NICE's partners' council is appointed by the Secretary of State and meets annually to review the annual report. It includes patients and representatives of patient organisations, professional organisations and healthcare industries.

www.nice.org.uk

But legal proceedings for medical injury are slow, complex and costly. They divert clinical staff from providing care, and can damage morale as well as public confidence. The system encourages defensiveness and secrecy, which hampers the NHS from learning and improving. Under the NHS Redress Act 2006, a scheme implemented in April 2007 provides an alternative to litigation for less severe cases. The Government hopes that the scheme will shift emphasis from attributing blame towards preventing harm, reducing risks and learning from mistakes. It does not fundamentally alter the existing legal system but provides an additional mechanism.

The intention is that the scheme should deal with claims under £20,000, avoiding the courts altogether; if a patient accepts compensation under the scheme, they will be barred from taking legal proceedings. Compensation is intended to be roughly equal to what a court might order. The Act applies only to NHS hospital care and excludes GP practices, dental surgeries and private healthcare. The NHS Litigation Authority will decide liability and compensation, as well as instituting and investigating claims. The scheme does not include an appeals process, but if a patient is dissatisfied with the outcome, they may begin legal proceedings.

The Act applies to England and contains framework powers for Wales only. The scheme cannot apply in Scotland or Northern Ireland.

Further information
NHS redress: improving the response to patients, DH, October 2005.
NHS redress: statement of policy, DH, November 2005.

Key organisations

National Patient Safety Agency
The role of the NPSA (created in 2001) is to co-ordinate efforts across England and Wales to report mistakes affecting patient safety and initiate preventive measures. Its 'national reporting and learning system' (NRLS) is the first of its kind worldwide. The NPSA also tries to promote an open and fair culture in the NHS, encouraging all healthcare staff to report incidents without undue fear of personal reprimand.

Key organisations continued

Since 2005 the NPSA's work has also encompassed:
- the safety aspects of hospital design, cleanliness and food (transferred from NHS Estates)
- ensuring research is carried out safely, through its responsibility for the Central Office for Research Ethics Committees
- helping local organisations address concerns about individual doctors' and dentists' performance through its responsibility for the National Clinical Assessment Service, which it absorbed following the review of arm's-length bodies (see page 16)
- managing contracts with the three confidential inquiries into patient outcome and death, maternal and child health, and suicide and homicide by mentally ill people – all transferred from NICE.

A review of the NPSA in 2006 recommended it should refocus on its core objective of collecting and analysing patient safety data, while the NRLS should be redesigned to make it easier for clinical staff to report adverse events confidentially without fear of retribution.
www.npsa.nhs.uk

NHS Litigation Authority

The NHSLA, set up in 1995, handles negligence claims against NHS bodies in England, and operates a risk management programme to help raise standards and reduce incidents leading to claims. It also monitors human rights case-law on the NHS's behalf.

In 2005/06 it received 5,697 claims for clinical negligence and paid out £560.3 million in damages and costs. Fewer than 50 clinical negligence cases a year are contested in court, and 96 per cent of the NHSLA's cases are settled out of court. Of all clinical claims handled since 1997:
- 38 per cent were abandoned by the claimant
- 43 per cent were settled out of court
- 4 per cent were settled in court
- 15 per cent are outstanding.

www.nhsla.com

Healthcare professions' responsibility for quality

Modernising professional self-regulation
NHS patients need to know that the staff who care for them are well-trained and competent. Professional self-regulation has been a cornerstone of the NHS since it began, yet events such as the Bristol Royal Infirmary inquiry, the Alder Hey cases – in which organs from dead children were retained without their families' knowledge – and Dr Harold Shipman's conviction for multiple murders highlighted the need for reform.

Professional self-regulation covers education, registration, training, continuing professional development and revalidation. It includes setting standards for deciding who should enter and remain members of a profession, and determining their fitness to practise. Its underpinning principles are:
- clarity about standards
- maintaining public confidence
- transparency in tackling fitness to practise
- responsiveness to and protection of patients.

The NHS Plan stipulated that regulatory bodies had to reform to become smaller, with much greater public and patient representation, faster, more transparent procedures and more meaningful accountability to the public and the health service. This was reinforced by the Kennedy Report on the Bristol Royal Infirmary inquiry a year later (see page 67). The Government has insisted that regulators develop common systems across the professions and agree standards that put patients' interests first. It is keen that self-regulation keeps pace with change in the NHS as well as society's attitudes and public opinion. Professional regulatory bodies must be open and make improvements based on feedback from patients, their representatives and the public. They must deal with complaints quickly, thoroughly, objectively and in a way that is responsive to the complainant while treating fairly the health professional complained against.

New regulatory bodies have been introduced for nursing, midwifery and health visiting and for the allied health professions:
- The Nursing and Midwifery Council replaced the UK Central Council in 2002 as the body responsible for governing nurses, midwives and health visitors.
- The Health Professions Council is responsible for the professions previously regulated by the Council for Professions Supplementary to Medicine, and

includes groups of healthcare professionals not previously covered by formal statutory regulation.
- The Council for Healthcare Regulatory Excellence (see page 92) oversees all the other professional regulatory bodies.

The General Medical Council is the regulatory body for doctors. A total of 4,980 complaints were lodged against doctors in 2005 – almost 100 a week. This compares with 1,000 (19 a week) in 1996.

Following the Shipman inquiry, the chief medical officer reviewed the regulation of the medical profession, and a parallel review of non-medical professional regulation also took place.

The Government subsequently published its proposals in a white paper, *Trust, assurance and safety: the regulation of health professionals in the 21st century*. Key changes include:
- making regulators more independent – for example, by professional members no longer forming the majority on regulatory bodies, and an independent adjudicator for doctors
- ensuring healthcare professionals are objectively revalidated throughout their career and remain up-to-date with clinical best practice
- moving from the criminal standard of proof to the civil standard with a sliding scale in fitness-to-practise cases
- a stronger role for the medical Royal Colleges
- a system of regional GMC affiliates to help local employers address concerns about doctors
- a comprehensive strategy for prevention, treatment and rehabilitation services for all health professionals.

At the same time the Government published its response to the final report of the Shipman inquiry. Key changes include:
- measures to ensure patients registering concerns are taken seriously
- more systematic use of information about the clinical outcomes of individual practitioners and teams
- bringing together information from different sources for a fuller picture about professionals
- all primary care organisations to adopt best practice in investigating and acting on concerns.

Further information

Trust, assurance and safety: the regulation of health professionals in the 21st century, DH, February 2007.

Learning from tragedy, keeping patients safe: overview of the Government's action programme in response to the recommendations of the Shipman Inquiry, DH, February 2007.

Good doctors, safer patients: proposals to strengthen the system to assure and improve the performance of doctors and to protect the safety of patients – a report by the chief medical officer, DH, July 2006.

Fifth report – safeguarding patients: lessons from the past – proposals for the future, Shipman Inquiry, December 2004.

General Medical Council: www.gmc-uk.org
Nursing and Midwifery Council: www.nmc-uk.org
Health Professions Council: www.hpc-uk.org

Key organisation: Council for Healthcare Regulatory Excellence

CHRE is a statutory body responsible to Parliament and independent of the Department of Health. It covers all the UK, promoting best practice and consistency in professional self-regulation in nine bodies:
- General Medical Council
- General Dental Council
- General Optical Council
- General Osteopathic Council
- General Chiropractic Council
- Health Professions Council
- Nursing and Midwifery Council
- Royal Pharmaceutical Society of Great Britain
- Pharmaceutical Society of Northern Ireland.

It has 19 members – one from each of the nine bodies and ten lay members. With parliamentary approval, CHRE can force a regulator to change its rules. It also has the power to refer unduly lenient decisions about professionals' fitness to practise to the High Court for review.
www.chre.org.uk

Continuing professional development

In *A first class service* (see page 84), the DH defined continuing professional development (CPD) as:

> a process of lifelong learning for all individuals and teams which meets the needs of patients and delivers the health outcomes and healthcare priorities of the NHS, and which enables professionals to expand and fulfil their potential.

In a climate of constant change, it is important that members of all professions demonstrate that they are keeping their knowledge and skills up to date: it is no longer sufficient simply to establish competence at the beginning of a career. Many professions, not just in healthcare, are beginning to adopt mandatory CPD. For individuals, CPD should:

- maintain professional competence and enable them, their teams and organisation to meet patients' needs, carry out their work with confidence and assist them in the event of an untoward incident
- provide them with the professional and personal satisfaction that they are working to the best of their ability and for the greater benefit of patients, colleagues and their employer
- help sustain motivation and interest in their work
- help meet career aspirations and learning needs, support flexible career pathways and allow them to take on wider responsibilities if necessary
- help them keep their jobs or enhance the possibility of finding another job
- help them identify the skills and knowledge they need to develop, preparing them for future opportunities.

CPD is as important for NHS organisations as it is for individuals. A professional's failure to keep up to date could have serious results, while allowing their skills and knowledge to become obsolete is to waste the investment in their education and training. In *Continuing professional development – quality in the new NHS* (July 1999) the DH stated that 'every health organisation needs to develop a locally managed, systematic approach to CPD'. The core principles are that CPD should be:

- purposeful and patient-centred
- participative, fully involving the individual and other relevant stakeholders
- targeted at identified educational need
- educationally effective

CPD: a four-part cyclical process

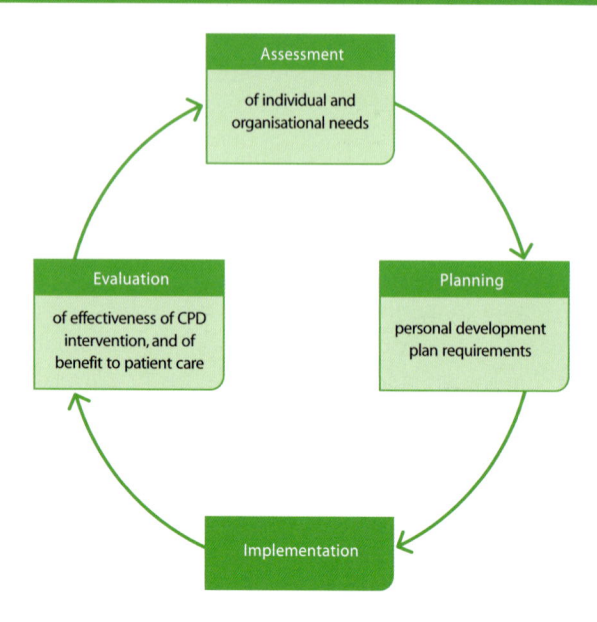

```
        Assessment
        of individual and
        organisational needs

Evaluation                      Planning
of effectiveness of CPD         personal development
intervention, and of            plan requirements
benefit to patient care

        Implementation
```

Source: *Continuing professional development,* Department of Health, 1999

- part of a wider organisational development plan supporting local and national service objectives
- focused on the development needs of clinical teams across traditional professional and service boundaries
- designed to build on previous knowledge, skills and experience
- designed to enhance the skills of interpreting and applying knowledge based on research and development.

As shown in the chart above, CPD is a cyclical process.

Code of conduct for NHS managers

Just as doctors, nurses and other health workers have codified ethics, so now do NHS managers. Written by senior managers in collaboration with the DH, the code states that all NHS managers must:

- make the care and safety of patients their first concern and act to protect them from risk
- respect the public, patients, relatives, carers, NHS staff and partners in other agencies
- be honest and act with integrity

- accept responsibility for their own work and the proper performance of the people they manage
- show their commitment to working as a team member by working with all their colleagues in the NHS and the wider community
- take responsibility for their own learning and development.

NHS organisations must incorporate the code in the contracts of chief executives and directors, and investigate alleged breaches. Those who break the code can be dismissed from the NHS and barred from re-employment within it.

Further information
Briefing 78: Managing for excellence in the NHS and the code of conduct for NHS managers, NHS Confederation, February 2003.

Feedback from patients

National patient surveys
Listening to patients' views is essential for a patient-centred health service. To deliver improvements, the NHS has to know what people need and expect from it, and how well they think the service has responded to their needs and expectations.

The programme of national patient surveys has three aims:
- to provide feedback for local quality improvement
- to assess users' experience for performance ratings, inspections and reviews
- to monitor patients' experience nationally.

The Healthcare Commission is responsible for carrying out national survey programmes. In 2006 it carried out surveys of diabetes patients and users of secondary mental health services. In 2007 it conducted its fourth survey of community mental health service users.

The DH launched the GP patient survey in 2006, which asked 5 million patients about their experiences of topics such as flexible booking, telephone access and opening hours. The results will be used to reward those GP practices offering patients good access to services.

Further information
GP patient survey: your doctor, your experience, your say – guidance for strategic health authorities, primary care trusts and GP practices, DH, November 2006.
Variations in the experiences of patients in England: analysis of the Healthcare Commission's 2003/2004 national surveys of patients, Healthcare Commission, October 2005.

Local patient surveys
The NHS Plan also requires each trust to obtain feedback from its own patients about their experiences of care. These surveys are intended to:
- track changes in patients' experience of trusts, year on year
- provide information for local quality improvement initiatives
- inform each trust's performance ratings and the performance indicators.

Trusts can seek support in carrying out their surveys from the NHS Patient Survey Programme Advice Centre.

Further information
Lost in translation: why are patients more satisfied with the NHS than the public? NHS Confederation, 2006.
NHS Patient Survey Programme Advice Centre: **www.nhssurveys.org**

Complaints

The NHS complaints procedure covers complaints about any matter connected with NHS services provided by NHS organisations or GPs, dentists, opticians and pharmacists. It also covers services provided overseas or by the private sector where the NHS has paid for them.

Every NHS organisation must have a well-defined mechanism for investigating and resolving complaints. It should be open, fair, flexible and conciliatory, and should encourage communication on all sides. It should also be well publicised. Complaints should be dealt with speedily and efficiently, and complainants should be treated courteously and sympathetically while being involved as far as possible in decisions about how their complaints are handled.

All NHS organisations must have a designated complaints manager, readily accessible to both the public and staff. They should be available to complainants who do not wish to raise their concerns with those directly involved with their care, or where frontline staff are unable to deal with the complaint. Complaints managers must have access to all relevant records, involve the complainant from the outset and keep them informed throughout the process. A senior person in the organisation – usually at board level – must take responsibility for the local complaints procedure.

Each organisation should establish a clear system to ensure investigations are carried out properly, and ensure appropriate conciliation or mediation services are available. A complaint can be made by a patient or person affected or likely to be affected by the actions or decisions of an NHS organisation or primary care practitioner. A complaint can also be made by someone acting on behalf of the patient or person, with their consent. It should normally be made within six months, though this can be waived if there is good reason for a delay. Complaints can be made orally or in writing, including e-mail.

Complaints may go through three stages, though most are expected to be settled at the first stage.

Local resolution
Complaints should be made first to the organisation or primary care practitioner providing the service. The aim is to resolve complaints quickly and as close to the source as possible. The complaints manager must send the complainant a written acknowledgement of the complaint within two working days. NHS bodies must seek to resolve all complaints within 20 working days. If this is not possible in complex cases, the complaints manager should agree a new date with the complainant. Finally, the complaints manager must prepare a written response that describes the investigation and summarises its conclusions. This must normally be signed by the chief executive. Foundation trusts may have their own arrangements.

Independent review
If a complainant is unhappy with the organisation's response, and local resolution has failed, they can ask the Healthcare Commission for an independent review. This also applies to foundations trusts.

Ombudsman

If a complainant remains unhappy after local resolution and independent review, he or she can complain to the Ombudsman (see page 100).

In the 2006 white paper, *Our health, our care, our say*, the Government announced it would develop 'a comprehensive single complaints system across health and social care' by 2009.

In 2005/06, NHS trusts received 95,047 complaints, a 5 per cent increase on the previous year. Three out of four were resolved locally within 20 days. Complaints included:
- 36,000 about all aspects of clinical care
- 11,500 about delays and cancellations of outpatient appointments
- 11,500 about the attitude of staff.

Independent Complaints Advocacy Services (ICAS)

Every trust and PCT has an ICAS to help individuals pursue complaints about the NHS. Complainants can contact their local ICAS office direct, or through complaints managers at hospitals and GP practices, NHS Direct, or the patient advice and liaison service. ICAS aims to ensure complainants have access to the support they need to articulate their concerns and navigate the complaints system. It can simply offer advice or write letters and attend meetings to speak on the complainant's behalf. Since 2006 three independent organisations with experience of advocacy have delivered ICAS under contract across England.

Further information
The first year of ICAS: 1 September 2003–31 August 2004, DH, January 2005.

Freedom of information

The Freedom of Information Act 2000 requires every public authority to adopt a 'publication scheme' that specifies the classes of information the authority publishes, the form it takes and whether it charges for the information. Each scheme must be approved by the Information Commissioner, an independent public official responsible for overseeing operation of the Act, who also has powers of enforcement.

Since January 2005, NHS organisations must answer requests for information within the terms of the individual right of access given by the Act. This applies to all types of recorded information held by the organisation regardless of its date, although the Act specifies some exemptions. Anyone making a request must be told whether the organisation holds the information and, if so, be supplied with it – generally within 20 working days. Organisations also have a duty to provide advice or help to anyone seeking information. Where a request for information is denied, it may be possible to appeal against the decision.

www.informationcommissioner.gov.uk
www.foi.nhs.uk

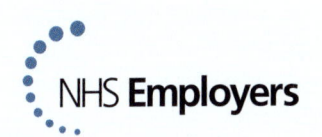

NHS Employers

The 2007 edition of **The healthy workplaces handbook** is your essential, all-encompassing NHS guide to health, safety and welfare in the workplace.

- 20 new chapters of concise, user-friendly, digestible information
- Accessible ring binder format
- Searchable online version
- Regular updates on the very latest regulations and requirements

Prices from £34.95

For more information please call 020 7074 3332 or email us at hwhandbook@nhsemployers.org

www.nhsemployers.org/hwhandbook

A part of the NHS Confederation working on behalf of the NHS

Key organisation: the Ombudsman

The office of the Parliamentary and Health Service Ombudsman (sometimes referred to as the Health Service Commissioner) undertakes independent investigations into complaints about the NHS in England, as well as Government departments and other public bodies. It is completely independent of the NHS and Government. In the NHS, the Ombudsman investigates complaints that a hardship or injustice has been caused by its failure to provide a service, by a failure in service or by maladministration. The Ombudsman looks into complaints against private health providers only if the treatment was funded by the NHS.

Complainants can only refer their cases to the Ombudsman after failing to achieve a resolution with the organisation or practitioner they are complaining against – for example, because of delays in dealing with a complaint locally or failure to get a satisfactory answer. The Ombudsman can consider complaints from a patient; a close member of the family, partner or representative, if the patient is unable to act for themselves; or from someone who has suffered injustice or hardship as a result of the actions of the NHS. A complaint will normally only be considered within a year of the events which gave rise to it.

The Ombudsman publishes detailed reports of investigations, which identify common themes in complaints. The reports are intended to be used as training tools to improve services, and chief executives are asked to ensure all clinical directors and complaints managers are aware of them. They are also considered by the House of Commons public administration committee.
www.ombudsman.org.uk

5

Financing the NHS

Sources of funding

Taxation
Funding healthcare through taxation ensures universal access to services irrespective of ability to pay. In 2006/07, 76.2 per cent of NHS funding in England came from general taxation – the Consolidated Fund – and 18.4 per cent from the NHS element of national insurance.

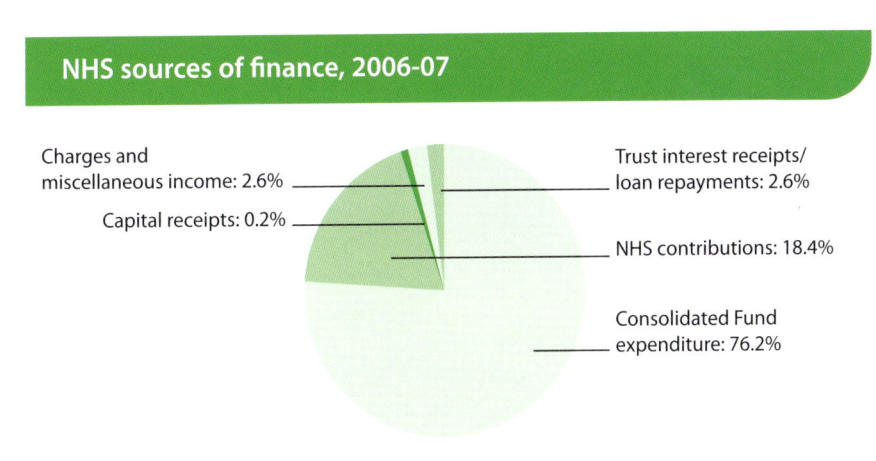

NHS sources of finance, 2006-07

- Charges and miscellaneous income: 2.6%
- Capital receipts: 0.2%
- Trust interest receipts/loan repayments: 2.6%
- NHS contributions: 18.4%
- Consolidated Fund expenditure: 76.2%

Source: Annual report 2006, Department of Health

101

Apart from social security payments, the health service is the biggest single item of public expenditure, absorbing 17 per cent of tax and national insurance contributions (NICs).

General taxation is generally regarded as being a highly efficient way of financing healthcare: it means the Government has both a strong incentive and the capacity to control costs; administrative costs especially tend to be low. As taxation draws revenue from a wide base, it helps minimise distortions in particular sectors of the economy. The social insurance element of NHS financing in the form of NICs paid by employees and employers, although relatively small, has been found to be highly progressive – that is, what people pay directly reflects what they can afford.

However, financing healthcare through taxation means the overall level of resources is constrained by what the Government judges the economy can afford and what is electorally viable, and choices between what services are and are not provided are made centrally. Many would argue that in the past the UK system has gone too far in controlling expenditure, leading to under-investment in the NHS compared with other countries over many years. The degree of individual choice available to patients has tended to be relatively limited.

Charges

The NHS currently charges for a limited number of clinical services – mainly prescriptions, dental treatments, sight tests, glasses and contact lenses. These out-of-pocket payments account for about 2 per cent of NHS funding. The principle remains that they should be paid only by those who can afford them, with a safety net built into the system so that those who cannot afford to pay do not have to and are not discouraged from seeking advice and treatment. A wide range of exemptions applies, including in most cases young and elderly people and those who are unemployed or on low incomes.

Further information

Third report of session 2005–06: NHS charges, House of Commons Health Committee, July 2006.

Prescriptions, dental treatment, sight tests

Since April 2007, prescription charges in England have been £6.85 per item. Prescription charges are set separately in Scotland and Northern Ireland. NHS Wales abolished prescription charges altogether in April 2007. It is estimated that about 50 per cent of the population of England does not have to pay prescription charges. In 2005, 87.6 per cent of prescription items were dispensed free to patients. Most courses of dental treatment cost £15.90 or £43.60, depending on their complexity. The maximum charge for complex dental treatment is £194. A sight test costs £18.39, although they have been free in Scotland since 2006. In addition, there are currently limited charges for non-clinical services such as single maternity rooms and car parking.

Recovering the costs of road accidents

Since the 1930s hospitals have been entitled by law to collect money for treating road traffic accident victims. A revised, centralised system for this was introduced in 1999, with the aim of streamlining collection of charges from drivers' insurance companies and setting a national tariff of charges to reflect the real costs of treatment.

NHS charges are levied when someone is involved in a road accident, is examined or treated at an NHS hospital and is then paid compensation for their injuries. The charges are paid by whoever pays the compensation, and raised £110 million for the NHS in England in 2006, £7.6 million in Scotland and £8 million in Wales. The money is paid direct to the hospitals that have provided the treatment. The Compensation Recovery Unit, part of the Benefits Agency, collects the charges, which are:
- flat rate for treatment without admission: £505
- daily rate for treatment with admission: £620
- maximum in any one case: £37,100.

In addition, since January 2007 the NHS has been able to recover costs from insurance companies for treating patients in all cases where personal injury compensation is paid. The injury costs recovery scheme is expected eventually to raise an extra £150 million a year in England, Wales and Scotland.

Overseas visitors

Anyone who is lawfully 'ordinarily resident' in the UK is entitled to free NHS treatment, regardless of nationality. British citizens who do not normally live in the UK may have to pay charges for NHS treatment, regardless of whether they have paid UK taxes and national insurance contributions, unless they are eligible for certain exemptions. British state pensioners who split their time between the UK and another European Economic Area member state are exempt from charges. Responsibility for deciding who is entitled to free treatment rests with the hospital providing the treatment. Asylum seekers whose application for refuge in the UK is outstanding are entitled to use NHS services without charge.

Other sources

Other sources of NHS funding come from land sales and income generation schemes. In addition, the Big Lottery Fund provides funding for health (as well as education and the environment). UK-wide, it has distributed £300 million to help set up healthy living centres, and given over £360 million for coronary heart disease, stroke and cancer services. It is also allocating £84 million for palliative care and support and information services for people with cancer and other life-threatening conditions.

Further information
www.biglotteryfund.org.uk

Resource allocation

The Treasury is responsible for overall public expenditure. Every two years it conducts a comprehensive spending review of all Government departments covering three years. After each review, the Department of Health – like all Government departments – draws up a public service agreement with the Treasury, setting out what it is expected to provide with its new resources over a three-year period. The DH in turn issues priorities and planning guidance to the NHS. The Treasury makes block grants to the Scottish Parliament, Welsh Assembly and the Northern Ireland Assembly, from which they allocate funds for the NHS.

Spending on the NHS divides into these main programmes:
- *hospital and community health services* (HCHS), and discretionary family health services. This covers hospital and community health services, prescribing costs

Vital statistics: NHS planned net spending 2007/08

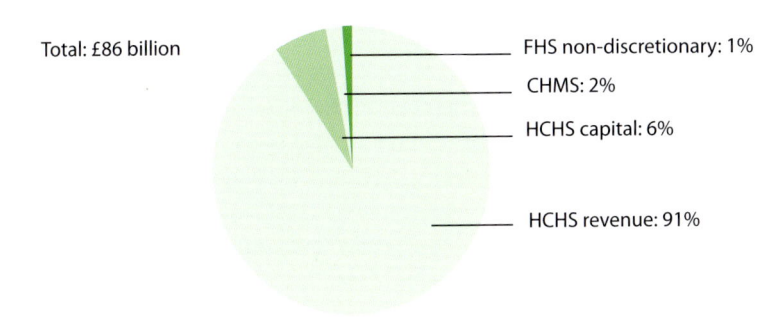

Total: £86 billion

FHS non-discretionary: 1%
CHMS: 2%
HCHS capital: 6%
HCHS revenue: 91%

Source: Department of Health

for drugs and appliances and discretionary general medical services (which include reimbursements of GMS GPs' practice staff, premises, out-of-hours and IT expenses). It also includes other centrally funded initiatives, services and special allocations managed centrally by the DH (such as education and training, and research and development).
- *non-discretionary family health services* (FHS). This covers demand-led family health services, including the remuneration of GPs for items such as capitation payments, health promotion and basic practice allowance, the cost of general dental and ophthalmic services, dispensing remuneration and income from dental and prescription charges.
- *central health and miscellaneous services* (CHMS), for example, certain public health functions and support to the voluntary sector.
- *administration of the Department of Health*.

Role of PCTs

Since 2003/04 the DH has made 'unified allocations' covering a three-year period direct to primary care trusts, which now control 85 per cent of the NHS budget. They have to plan the use of their resources over the three years as agreed with their strategic health authority. However, they must manage within their annual resource limit total for each year, although they can carry forward planned underspends of up to 0.25 per cent. These unified budget allocations cover:
- commissioning hospital, mental health and learning disability services
- providing community services
- PCT running costs
- GP and community nurses' prescribing costs
- primary care infrastructure.

Provided they are achieving the targets in their local delivery plan and keep sufficient in reserve to pay GPs, PCTs can use their resources as they see fit.

PCTs are responsible for funding the healthcare of all patients registered with GPs in their area. Under practice-based commissioning, PCTs delegate budgets to GP practices to commission acute, community and emergency care. PCTs' and practices' agreements with providers – NHS trusts, foundation trusts and, increasingly, independent providers – may no longer set activity levels, which are now decided by patient choice and funded through payment by results. However, all contracts and agreements do contain planned activity levels profiled across the year.

NHS trusts derive most of their income by providing services in this way, although they also earn some by providing private healthcare and are funded separately for training health professionals. They may also generate some income from shops or car parks on hospital premises.

NHS trusts and PCTs have to publish their costs for individual procedures on a consistent basis in the national schedule of reference costs. This gives details of the unit costs for a range of procedures and treatments, from x-rays to lung transplant surgery and from a visit by a district nurse to a home delivery by a midwife. Commissioners can use the information when negotiating agreements, and identify areas for improving efficiency.

Further information
2006–07 and 2007–08 primary care trusts' revenue allocations: a short guide, DH, July 2005.

Weighted capitation formula

A weighted capitation formula is used to determine each PCT's target share of resources. This reflects the age distribution of a PCT's population and the health needs it may have due to deprivation or high mortality and morbidity levels, as well as unavoidable geographical variations in the cost of providing services. The intention is that every PCT should be able to commission similar levels of health services for populations in similar need.

The formula's components and their relative weights are:
- hospital and community health services (77 per cent)
- prescribing (13 per cent)
- primary medical services (9 per cent)
- HIV/AIDS (1 per cent).

These components are used to adjust each PCT's 'crude population' based on 2001 census estimates. Some PCTs will currently be funded above their target level and others below it (this is known as their distance from target), reflecting the legacy of previous years' allocations. Ministers decide for each allocation round the level of increase that all PCTs receive in order to deliver on national and local priorities and the level of extra resources to PCTs that are under target, to move them closer to their weighted capitation targets. It is intended that no PCT will be more than 3.5 per cent under target by the end of 2007/08.

Further information
Resource allocation: weighted capitation formula: fifth edition, DH, May 2005.

Resource accounting and budgeting

Resource accounting and budgeting (RAB) was introduced as the financial management framework in the public sector in 2001, and the DH applied its principles to the NHS. This meant that if a trust reported a deficit in one year, its income was reduced by that amount the following year. In addition, the trust's in-year deficit appeared on its balance sheet and was carried forward to future years, giving a cumulative position. This cumulative position was used to assess whether the trust had achieved its statutory duty to 'break even taking one year with another'. The combination of a cumulative deficit and income reduction the following year was often referred to as a 'double deficit'.

The Audit Commission found RAB had been applied inconsistently, preventing trusts from planning ahead and worsening deficits. It recommended that RAB be abolished in the NHS and deductions returned. The DH acknowledged in the *NHS operating framework for 2007/08*: 'The way in which RAB is applied to NHS trusts... will become increasingly unsustainable,' and it announced at the end of March 2007 that RAB would be abolished.

Further information
Learning the lessons from financial failure in the NHS, Audit Commission, July 2006.

Spotlight on policy: payment by results

Far-reaching changes have been made to the way money flows through the NHS in England between commissioners and providers. A system of payment by results has been introduced in an attempt to ensure funding follows the patient. This is designed to underpin Government policy on increasing patient choice and encourage a diversity of providers. The changes are being implemented gradually over five years to 2008.

The aim is to provide a transparent system for paying trusts which encourages activity to reduce waiting times. PCTs commission the volume of activity they require for their populations, but instead of drawing up block agreements with NHS trusts as previously, the trusts and other providers are paid for the activity they undertake. A tariff derived from national reference costs removes prices from local negotiation, so that commissioners focus instead on gains in patient choice, quality, shorter waiting time, volumes of activity and efficiency.

The DH has issued a code of conduct for payment by results to establish core principles, ground rules for organisational behaviour and expectations of how the system should operate – as well as to minimise disputes.

Early experience has shown the impact of payment by results on an organisation to be much faster than envisaged. It has a significant effect on people and culture, and exposes fragilities in the system. The DH acknowledges that in combination with other reforms, payment by results 'represents very powerful chemistry'. Errors in the tariff for 2006/07 led to its temporary withdrawal early in 2006. A subsequent review of the tariff-setting process recommended more transparency, greater involvement of frontline clinicians and managers, piloting of new tariffs and earlier indication of the next year's tariff. As a result, no substantial changes were made to the scope and structure of the tariff for 2007/08.

Further information
Report on the tariff setting process for 2006/07: Lawlor report, DH, July 2006.
Code of conduct for payment by results, DH, January 2006.
Reforming NHS financial flows: introducing payment by results, DH, October 2002.

Capital

Reforming capital investment

Until 2007 the DH allocated operational capital to NHS trusts and PCTs according to a formula, and distributed strategic capital to SHAs based on weighted capitation. It has now replaced this system with a borrowing regime similar to that which already applied to foundation trusts. The DH was concerned that under the old system, capital could be allocated to organisations that attracted insufficient revenue through patient choice to service the capital charges resulting from the investment. It also identified a risk that NHS trusts could develop investment plans that proved to be incompatible with a prudential borrowing limit, and so create an obstacle to their becoming foundation trusts. The new system is intended to prevent cash leaking from capital to revenue. Therefore, from 2007/08, access to capital funding is decided by the affordability of proposed investments and financed by loans and borrowing subject to a prudential borrowing regime.

However, arrangements for PCTs remain the same. In 2007/08 they will receive £382 million in capital, allocated as (figures rounded up):
- £167 million operational capital for maintaining and modernising buildings and replacing equipment (24 per cent increase on 2006/07)
- £156 million strategic capital to fund new equipment and buildings (29 per cent increase)
- £60 million to modernise dental premises and equipment (50 per cent increase).

Private finance initiative (PFI)

PFI involves a public–private partnership between an NHS organisation and a private sector consortium that makes private capital available for health service projects. All major NHS capital projects are expected to consider whether PFI could represent a value-for-money solution.

The private sector consortium will usually include a construction company, a funding organisation and a facilities management provider. Contracts for major PFI schemes may be for 30 years or more and are typically DBFO (design, build, finance and operate) projects. This means the private sector partner is responsible for:
- designing the facilities (based on the requirements specified by the NHS)
- building the facilities (to time and at a fixed cost)

- financing the capital cost (with the return to be recovered through continuing to make the facilities available and meeting NHS requirements)
- operating the facilities (providing facilities management and other support services).

PFI schemes must demonstrate value for money, which is usually achieved by the PFI partner assuming risks which would otherwise have been borne by the public sector, and by efficiency savings. The PFI contract sets out the performance standards required of the consortium. The NHS makes no payments until services are provided to the agreed standard, and then they must be maintained to ensure full payment.

The aims of PFI are to increase innovation and reduce the overall risks associated with procuring new assets and services for the NHS, as well as to improve the quality and cost-effectiveness of public services. Because the PFI partner's capital is at risk, they have an incentive to perform well throughout the life of the contract, while private sector management, commercial and creative skills are harnessed for the NHS's benefit.

Critics have questioned whether PFI will really provide long-term value for money for the NHS, and have claimed services have been cut in some cases to make schemes affordable. In response the Government has said: 'PFI is only a procurement tool – not an end in itself – and will only be used in cases where it offers value for money to the taxpayer and the NHS.' It is not advised in projects involving rapid change, such as IT. As the NHS is undergoing a period of rapid change, it can be argued that PFI will need to adapt to accommodate the changes.

The launch of the Treasury report, *PFI: strengthening long-term partnerships*, confirmed the Government's commitment to a PFI investment programme for public services and describes the steps it is taking to strengthen PFI with measures to increase flexibility and reinforce the requirement for value for money.

By early 2007, 84 hospitals had been built under PFI, 25 were under construction and seven other projects had been approved.

Further information
PFI: strengthening long-term partnerships, HM Treasury, March 2006.

NHS Local Improvement Finance Trust (LIFT)
NHS LIFT aims to encourage investment in primary care and community-based facilities and services to achieve the NHS Plan target of 500 one-stop primary care centres and the refurbishment or replacement of up to 3,000 GP premises. It is similar to PFI, except that it is a joint venture between PCTs, the private sector partner, local authorities and GPs.

Partnerships for Health, a public–private partnership between the DH and Partnerships UK, was set up to invest money in NHS LIFT and help attract additional private funding; the DH became the sole owner in 2006.

By early 2007, 100 new GP premises had been built under the LIFT programme, with a further 79 under construction. NHS LIFT seeks investment in primary care developments by bundling them together. So far, 49 local LIFT schemes are renting accommodation to GPs, pharmacists, opticians, dentists and others on a lease basis. The latest wave of schemes add the option to include clinical and facilities management services as well as buildings and maintenance. The total value of the LIFT programme is £1.2 billion.

Further information
Innovation in the NHS: local improvement finance trusts, National Audit Office, May 2005.

NHS spending

The era of growth
From the time the NHS was founded until the end of the 1990s, its annual average increase in funding was just over 3 per cent – slightly more than the real growth in the economy as a whole. However, from the early 1980s, real spending changes were erratic. Taking into account the level of inflation in the NHS rather than in the general economy, annual average growth was about 0.9 per cent from 1983 to 1987, 2 per cent from 1987 to 1992 and 1.4 per cent from 1992 to 1997. In 2000 the Government announced its intention to raise the share of national income spent on health to the European average: it then ranked 14th out of the 15 EU countries.

Vital statistics: UK health spending as a percentage of GDP

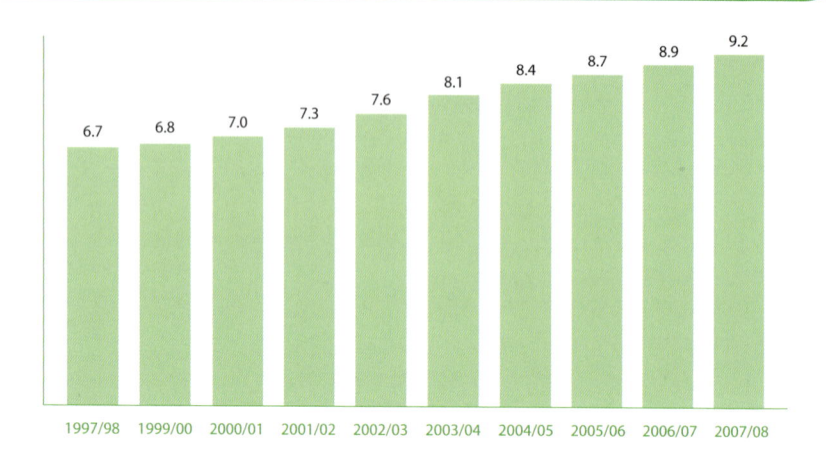

Year	%
1997/98	6.7
1999/00	6.8
2000/01	7.0
2001/02	7.3
2002/03	7.6
2003/04	8.1
2004/05	8.4
2005/06	8.7
2006/07	8.9
2007/08	9.2

Source: HM Treasury

In 2001 Derek Wanless was commissioned to produce the first evidence-based assessment of the NHS's long-term resource requirements (see opposite). As a result, the 2002 Budget heralded major increases in NHS spending until 2007/08: it is set to rise from £53.5 billion to £87.1 billion. These are the largest sustained increases in any five-year period in NHS history: an annual average increase of 7.4 per cent in real terms between 2002/03 and 2007/08, a total increase of 43 per cent in real terms over the period. This translates into a rise in NHS spending per household from £2,370 in 2001/02 to £4,060 in 2007/08. The aim is to put the NHS on a 'sound long-term financial footing', making significant investment in IT, buildings and equipment. It will also raise NHS spending to the EU average. To help pay for these increases, national insurance contributions were raised by 1 per cent from April 2003.

Derek Wanless produced a similar report for NHS Wales in 2003 (see page 188), while in Northern Ireland the Appleby Report of 2005 (see page 201) sought to predict future needs and resources.

Has the NHS given value for money?
Clinical outcomes, waiting times and patient satisfaction have all improved, while many other productivity gains are still working their way through the system. The true picture can be clouded by measures that often do not accurately reflect what the NHS does and confuse quality improvements with a loss of productivity.

Key text: Wanless Report

In 2001 the Chancellor commissioned Derek Wanless, former chief executive of the NatWest Bank, to examine demand and cost pressures in the NHS over the next 20 years and recommend the spending needed for a 'publicly funded, comprehensive, high-quality service available on the basis of clinical need and not ability to pay'. The Wanless review team published an interim report for consultation in November 2001 and its final report in April 2002.

Wanless found that although an ageing population would be an important influence, this would not be the main factor driving up costs. Patients were likely to demand more choice and higher-quality services. Improving information and communication technology would be key to achieving this, while the NHS would have to change its skill-mix and ways of working, and enhance the role of primary care.

Wanless concluded that spending would need to rise to between 9.4 per cent and 11.3 per cent of GDP by 2021, with the fastest growth before 2008. He warned: 'Both additional resources and radical reform are vital: neither would succeed without the other.'

Wanless's figures assume that plans for huge expansion of the workforce are achieved, that IT spend can be doubled and used productively while the NHS fulfils commitments on waiting times and national service frameworks. If productivity improvement falls short of 2 per cent a year, spending will need to rise to an even higher proportion of GDP.

His review endorsed decentralising the NHS, and argued that targets 'should be used with care'. There should be stability and certainty of funding, taking account of local needs without creating perverse incentives. He called too for greater transparency and better understanding of healthcare costs.

Securing our future: taking a long-term view. Final report, HM Treasury, April 2002.
www.hm-treasury.gov.uk

> **Key organisation: NHS Bank**

The NHS Bank was set up in 2003/04 as a mutual organisation serving the strategic health authorities. Its main functions include:
- responsibility for managing brokerage across the public capital programme, working with SHAs to manage the profile of capital expenditure
- co-ordinating cash brokerage across SHAs
- assisting in managing central budgets
- advising the DH on the financial impact of new policy developments.

However, despite unprecedented funding levels, the NHS in England overspent by £512 million in 2005/06, following a comparable overspend of £216 million the previous year. This represents 0.8 per cent of its £66.6 billion revenue in a year when its resources increased by 9.1 per cent. The overspend arose from deficits totalling £1.277 million and surpluses of £765 million. The worst financial problems were concentrated in the east and south-east of England. A mere 11 per cent of all organisations accounted for 70 per cent of the deficit. Most NHS organisations improved their services substantially and remained within budget.

PCTs spent their extra resources in 2005/06 on:
- secondary care – 53.3 per cent
- primary care – 27.5 per cent
- pay – 5.7 per cent
- supplies and services – 1.8 per cent
- debt repayment – 2.3 per cent
- other – 9.3 per cent.

NHS trusts spent their extra resources in 2005/06 on:
- pay – 56 per cent
- supplies and services, including drug costs – 33 per cent
- debt repayment – 5 per cent
- other – 6 per cent.

No single cause underlies the financial problems. There is little correlation between the size of an organisation's deficit and its allocation per head, nor with its performance rating. No evidence suggests organisations need to overspend to improve access to services. But deficits are concentrated in organisations that overspent in the previous year, suggesting that if they fail to address problems immediately they will find it increasingly difficult to recover their position.

The Government expects the NHS to return to financial balance in 2006/07 and to make a surplus of at least £250 million in 2007/08.

Further information
First report of session 2006–07: NHS deficits, House of Commons Health Committee, December 2006.
Briefing 135: Learning the lessons from financial failure in the NHS, NHS Confederation, September 2006.
Explaining NHS deficits 2003/04–2005/06: chief economist's report on NHS deficits, DH, February 2007.

Where the money is spent
NHS total net expenditure (revenue and capital) in England in 2006/07 was expected to be over £84.4 billion. The largest part of NHS spending is on hospital and community health services, discretionary family health services and related services. For 2006/07, planned net revenue expenditure for hospital, community and family health services is £76.6 billion and planned net capital expenditure is £5.2 billion.

The domination of spending on acute services reflects the demand for emergency treatment, and the continuing emphasis on reducing waiting lists and waiting times. Healthcare for people over 65 accounts for 43 per cent of the total expenditure.

Vital statistics: how hospital and community health services (HCHS) spending is divided

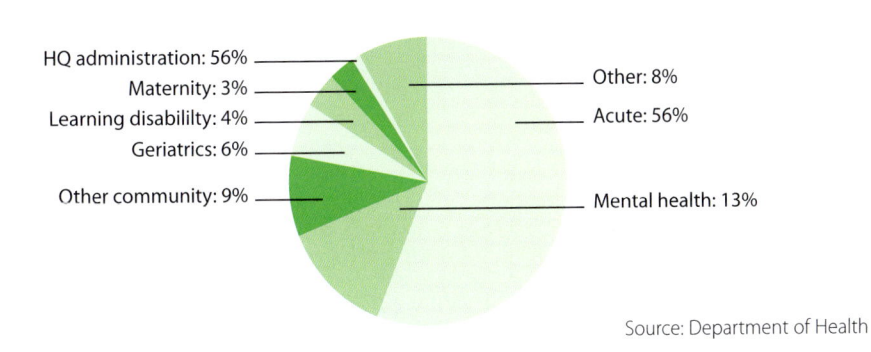

HQ administration: 56%
Maternity: 3%
Learning disabililty: 4%
Geriatrics: 6%
Other community: 9%
Other: 8%
Acute: 56%
Mental health: 13%

Source: Department of Health

The NHS in the UK 2007/08

Efficiency savings

Spending increases usually come with caveats about the level of efficiency savings the NHS is expected to make. It is expected to make efficiency gains of 2.5 per cent in 2007/08. Efficiency and productivity vary across the NHS, and the Government argues that significant benefits could come from trusts following best practice. The six main areas targeted for improved efficiency are:

Disposition of NHS resources 2006/07

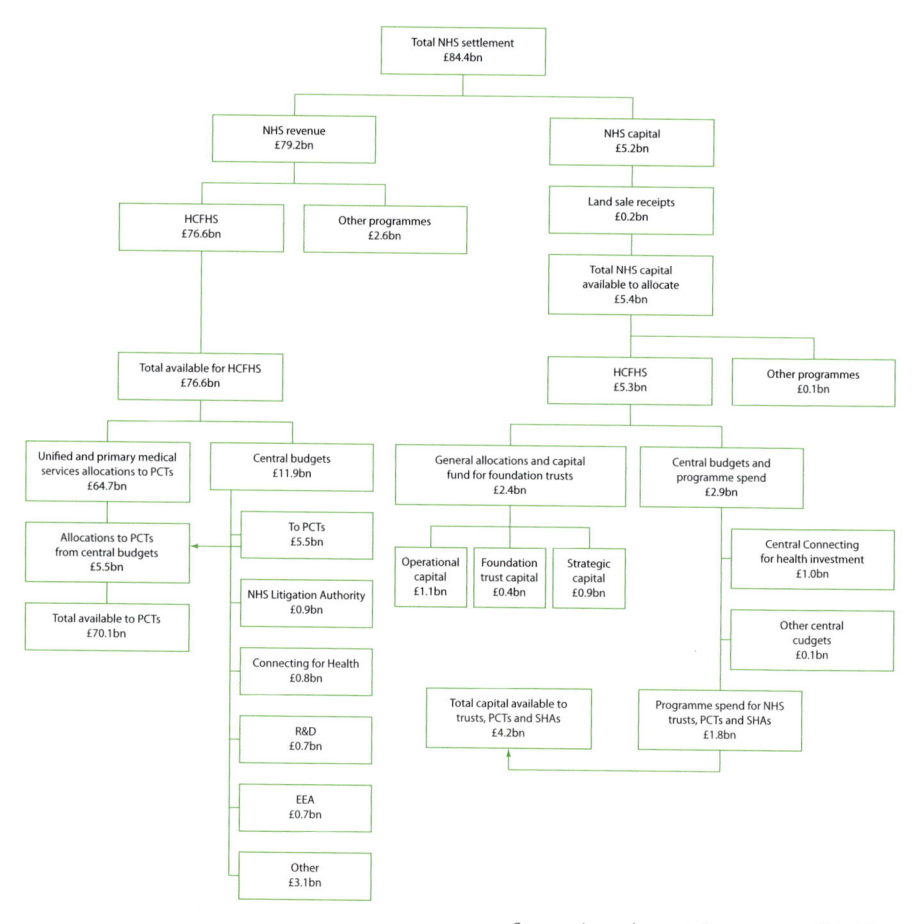

- Total NHS settlement £84.4bn
  - NHS revenue £79.2bn
    - HCFHS £76.6bn
      - Total available for HCFHS £76.6bn
        - Unified and primary medical services allocations to PCTs £64.7bn
          - Allocations to PCTs from central budgets £5.5bn
          - Total available to PCTs £70.1bn
        - Central budgets £11.9bn
          - To PCTs £5.5bn
          - NHS Litigation Authority £0.9bn
          - Connecting for Health £0.8bn
          - R&D £0.7bn
          - EEA £0.7bn
          - Other £3.1bn
    - Other programmes £2.6bn
  - NHS capital £5.2bn
    - Land sale receipts £0.2bn
    - Total NHS capital available to allocate £5.4bn
      - HCFHS £5.3bn
        - General allocations and capital fund for foundation trusts £2.4bn
          - Operational capital £1.1bn
          - Foundation trust capital £0.4bn
          - Strategic capital £0.9bn
        - Total capital available to trusts, PCTs and SHAs £4.2bn
        - Central budgets and programme spend £2.9bn
          - Central Connecting for health investment £1.0bn
          - Other central cudgets £0.1bn
          - Programme spend for NHS trusts, PCTs and SHAs £1.8bn
      - Other programmes £0.1bn

Source: Annual report, Department of Health

Vital statistics: health spending 2006/07

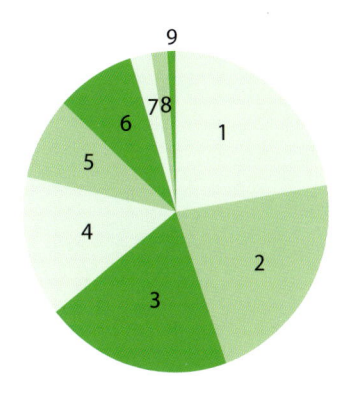

1. Urgent and emergency care: £13.7 billion
2. 'First contact' services – GPs, pharmacies, NHS Direct etc: £13.5 billion
3. Elective care – including day cases and outpatients: £12.1 billion
4. Community and intermediate care services: £8.6 billion
5. Specialised services: £5 billion
6. Mental health services: £5 billion
7. Maternity care: £1.3 billion
8. Promotion/prevention: £1 billion
9. Support for self-care: £500 million

Source: Department of Health

- potential for sharing corporate services
- procurement of outside services
- restructuring of the DH and arm's-length bodies
- reduction in the DH central budget to recycle funds to the front line
- improved commissioning of social care services
- Productive Time – a programme to maximise time spent by clinical, managerial and administrative staff on improving services: 'working smarter, not harder'.

In particular, the DH has identified £2.2 billion of savings from productivity improvements in:
- reducing variation in length of stay – £975 million
- reducing emergency admissions – £348 million
- reducing variation in outpatient referrals – £278 million
- managing surgical thresholds – £73 million
- increasing rates of day case procedures – £16 million
- reducing pre-operative bed days – £510 million.

Measuring inflation

Increases in the cost of goods and services used by the NHS are measured by the health service cost index (HSCI). The HSCI weights together price increases for a broad range of items – for example: drugs, medical equipment, fuel and telephone charges. Calculations are based on spending on these items reported in financial returns. Between 1992 and 2000, net NHS expenditure increased by 43 per cent in cash terms, by 17.4 per cent when inflation in the economy as a whole was taken into account and by 14.1 per cent after accounting for NHS-specific inflation.

Vital statistics: finished consultant episodes*

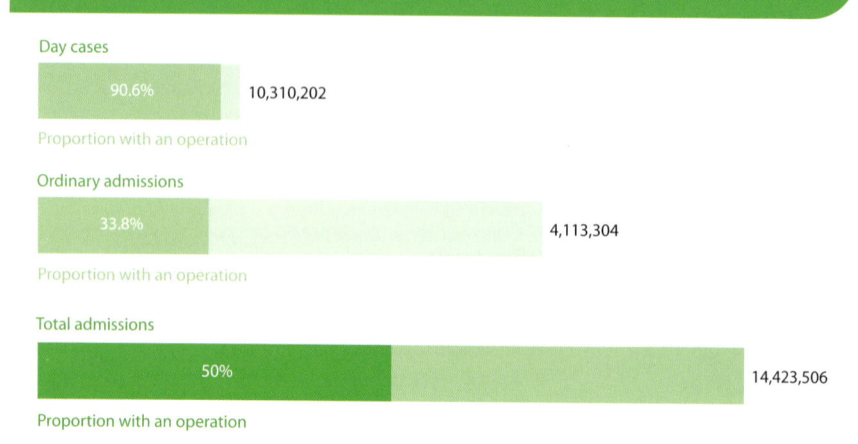

Day cases
90.6% — 10,310,202
Proportion with an operation

Ordinary admissions
33.8% — 4,113,304
Proportion with an operation

Total admissions
50% — 14,423,506
Proportion with an operation

* A finished consultant episode represents the completion of a patient's period of care under a consultant, after which they are either discharged or transferred to another consultant.

Source: The Information Centre

NHS Shared Business Services

NHS Shared Business Services was launched as a joint venture between the DH and the private sector company Xansa in 2005, building on an earlier shared financial services initiative that used two purpose-built centres in Leeds and Bristol. The intention is that SBS provides high-quality, cost-effective business services such as processing financial transactions, so that frontline organisations can concentrate on patient care. It currently provides finance, accounting and payroll services to over 100 NHS organisations, including PCTs, ambulance trusts, mental health trusts and non-departmental public bodies.
www.sbs.nhs.uk

Buying goods and services

Pharmaceutical Price Regulation Scheme (PPRS)

The PPRS regulates the prices of branded medicines and the profits that manufacturers are allowed to make on their sales to the NHS. It is a voluntary agreement made between the DH and the Association of the British Pharmaceutical Industry. A series of voluntary agreements has limited branded medicine prices and profits since 1957, each lasting five years or so.

Agreements cover all licensed, branded prescription medicines sold to the NHS. They do not cover products without a brand name (generics) nor over-the-counter branded products except when prescribed by a doctor. The PPRS is a UK-wide scheme, and covers around 80 per cent by value of the medicines used in the NHS in both primary and secondary care. The total NHS drugs bill in England was £11 billion in 2005/06, including both branded and generic medicines and drugs prescribed in the community as well as in hospital. Net expenditure on branded medicines in the community was £5.3 billion.

The PPRS seeks to achieve reasonable prices for the NHS, while recognising that the industry needs to earn the money to enable it to develop and market new and improved medicines. The agreement beginning in 2005 has secured for the NHS a 7 per cent price reduction for branded prescription medicines, which will save it more than £1.8 billion over the next five years. It requires companies to seek the DH's agreement for price increases. Those with NHS sales of more than £25 million a year must submit annual data on sales, costs, assets and profitability and repay the excess where profits exceed the agreed return on capital.

A maximum price scheme for generics – on which the NHS spends £1 billion a year – was introduced in 2000 to restrain the drugs bill after steep price rises, saving around £330 million a year. Since 2004, where there is a limited number of manufacturers of a generic medicine or the supply is concentrated, manufacturers have to seek the DH's agreement to any price increase. Manufacturers and wholesalers must submit quarterly information on income revenues, cost of purchases and volumes of transactions.

However, the Office of Fair Trading has claimed that the NHS is still paying too much for branded medicines and could save a further £500 million through far-reaching reforms to the PPRS and by making greater use of generic medicines.

Further information
Pharmaceutical Price Regulation Scheme: ninth report to Parliament, DH, July 2006.
PPRS market study report, OFT, February 2007.

Key organisations

NHS Purchasing and Supply Agency
This agency is responsible for ensuring the NHS gets the best value for money when purchasing other goods and services. It acts as a centre of expertise and knowledge in purchasing and supply matters, and contracts on a national basis for products and services which are strategically critical to the NHS. It also acts where large-scale purchasing power will yield greater savings than those achieved by contracting on a local or regional basis. PASA works with 400 NHS organisations and manages 3,000 national purchasing contracts, influencing around half the £7 billion the NHS spends on goods and services.

Part of PASA has been merged with NHS Logistics to create NHS Supply Chain, which will specialise in the supply and delivery of healthcare-related products and be managed by a private company.
www.pasa.doh.gov.uk

NHS Business Services Authority
This special health authority was set up in April 2006 to be the main processing facility for payment, reimbursement, remuneration and reconciliation for NHS patients, employees and others. It was formed from the Dental Practice Board, NHS Pensions Agency and the Prescription Pricing Authority.
www.nhsbsa.uk

NHS Counter Fraud Service
The NHS Counter Fraud Service was established to tackle fraud and corruption throughout the NHS, whether involving professionals, staff, patients or contractors. The service has more than 500 trained and accredited counter-fraud specialists throughout the NHS. Since 2000 it is estimated to have saved £811 million. Fraud by NHS professionals has fallen by up to 60 per cent and fraud by patients by 55 per cent since 1998. The NHS fraud and corruption reporting line is 0800 028 4060.
www.cfsms.nhs.uk

6

Staffing and human resources

As the UK's largest employer – indeed, one of the largest employers in the world – the NHS attaches special importance to good human resources policy and practice. Staff costs account for about 75 per cent of hospital expenditure. Effective recruitment, retention and remuneration of a well-trained and well-motivated workforce are seen as crucial factors in achieving the Government's ambitions for patient care.

Workforce planning

Current arrangements for NHS workforce planning are in a state of change. The Department of Health is drawing up its overall workforce strategy for the next five years, and arrangements for how NHS training is commissioned are under review. Strategic health authorities will have overall responsibility for workforce planning in their area, and will need to involve local employers. The Workforce Review Team currently advises the NHS on an annual basis on staffing needs and the need for training commissions.

Staff numbers

The NHS workforce has grown significantly since 1997, but this period of expansion appears to be coming to an end. Almost all the staffing targets in the NHS Plan have been achieved, and the NHS now intends to stabilise its workforce.

Vital statistics: NHS staff (whole-time equivalent)

Total: 1.3 million
Professionally-qualified clinical staff
1. Nurses: 29.6%
2. Scientific, therapeutic and technical: 9.9%
3. Doctors: 9%
4. Ambulance staff: 1.3%

Support to clinical staff
5. Support to doctors and nurses: 22.7%
6. Support to scientific, therapeutic and technical staff: 4.1%
7. Support to ambulance staff: 0.7%

NHS infrastructure support
8. Central functions: 7.7%
9. Hotel, property and estates: 5.5%
10. Managers and senior managers: 2%
11. Others 7.5%

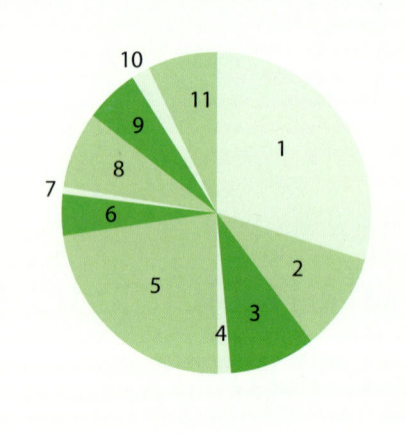

Source: The Information Centre

Financial pressures, administrative reorganisation and the need to clear historical deficits have had a major impact on NHS staff numbers, and the workforce is expected to fall. Around 1,500 compulsory redundancies have been declared out of a workforce of 1.3 million. The NHS is also facing a major challenge to employ the current cohort of nursing and other graduates.

Further information
Briefing 21: Consulting on proposed NHS redundancy arrangements, NHS Employers, August 2006.
Delivering the NHS Improvement Plan: the workforce contribution, DH, November 2004.
Staff in the NHS 2005, The Information Centre, April 2006.

Measuring workforce needs
The NHS National Workforce Projects' role is to support NHS organisations to achieve their workforce objectives and overcome the challenges that may prevent them having the right people in the right roles in the future. This means ensuring the NHS is able to plan for future workforce needs and can adapt to new ways of working.

Key organisation: NHS Employers

NHS Employers is the arm of the NHS Confederation responsible for workforce and employment issues on behalf of NHS organisations in England.

Set up by the DH in 2004, NHS Employers ensures the service itself drives the workforce agenda. It represents employers' views and acts on their behalf in the current priority areas of:
- pay and negotiations
- planning and workforce
- productivity
- 'employer of excellence'
- HR policy and practice.

The DH decided the broad framework within which NHS Employers operates, but employers themselves drive the organisation's agenda. Its policy board, with members drawn from a diverse range of organisations and professions, plays an important part in deciding on the work, position and direction of the organisation. More than 500 health service representatives have direct involvement in the design and delivery of its work through working groups, email reference groups and forums.

NHS Employers has conducted reviews of the NHS pension scheme and the GMS contract, terms and conditions for staff and associate specialist grade doctors and a new system of unsocial hours payments for staff. It has helped organisations on the full range of workforce issues as well as representing them nationally and internationally.

Further information
Annual review, NHS Employers, January 2007.
www.nhsemployers.org

The Workforce Review Team (WRT) produces data and intelligence about future workforce needs, reviewing in detail supply and demand and advising on the most practical and effective use of resources. It supplies information and advice to strategic health authorities and their workforce development directorates, commissioning and workforce planning leads, the DH, national workforce programme boards and individual trusts.

Further information
Workforce recommendations 2007/08, NHS Workforce Review Team, October 2006.
www.healthcareworkforce.nhs.uk

NHS Careers
NHS Careers is a service providing information on careers in the NHS in England. It consists of a 24-hour helpline, website, literature and supporting services for NHS employers, schools, colleges and careers advisers. Launched in 1999, it aims to make the workforce of the future aware of the 300 careers the NHS offers.
www.nhscareers.nhs.uk

Training

Training places have been increased since 1999 as part of the strategy to expand staff numbers. For example, the number of nurse graduates will continue to increase over the next year to 19,737 and then stabilise. The number of medical graduates also continues to rise and there is some potential for oversupply in the longer term, although graduates are currently entitled to a place on the foundation programme. The NHS will also need to respond to the recommendations of the Leitch review on skills for support staff.

Current arrangements for funding medical and other education in the NHS are complex and based on a historical model which is now under review. Responsibility for medical education is divided between the General Medical Council for undergraduate education, the Postgraduate Medical Education and Training Board (PMETB) for postgraduate education, and the deaneries which oversee the placing of students in their training placements within hospitals.

Vital statistics: medical school intake

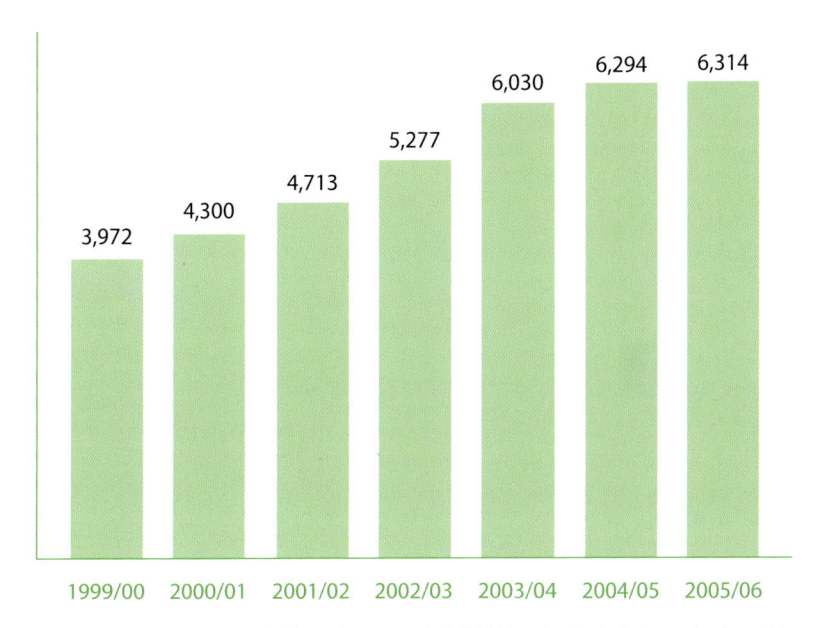

Year	Intake
1999/00	3,972
2000/01	4,300
2001/02	4,713
2002/03	5,277
2003/04	6,030
2004/05	6,294
2005/06	6,314

The figures above cover only English higher education institutions, and are for medicine only.
Source: Higher Education Funding Council for England

The 14 medical Royal Colleges and their faculties help define and monitor education and training, support doctors in their practice, and advise the Government, public and the profession on healthcare issues. Their representative body is the Academy of Medical Royal Colleges.

The Postgraduate Medical Education and Training Board, set up in 2003, brings together responsibility for all postgraduate medical education and assesses doctors who are completing final postgraduate training. It also oversees dental vocational training.

Further information
Briefing 19: The Postgraduate Medical Education and Training Board – what it means for the NHS, NHS Employers, May 2006.
Postgraduate Medical Education and Training Board **www.pmetb.org.uk**

Spotlight on policy: Modernising Medical Careers

The Modernising Medical Careers (MMC) project aims, through a major reform of postgraduate medical education, to develop competent doctors who are skilled at communicating and working as effective members of a team. As a key part of this, MMC is implementing significant changes to the medical career structures.

All graduates leaving medical school now enter a two-year foundation programme, designed to provide a solid grounding in practical medicine and develop core clinical skills. Integral to this, doctors are also required to enhance their communication, team-working and IT skills. This foundation training means they have an opportunity to develop experience in a range of specialties, and gain insight into possible career options or build a wider appreciation of medicine before embarking on specialist training. Importantly, for the first time, they must demonstrate their abilities and competence against explicit national standards set out in a curriculum.

At the end of the foundation programme, trainees will be ready to apply to enter specialty training (including general practice) and continue their career development. Under MMC, specialty training following the foundation programme has become competency-based, more focused and streamlined. The senior house officer and specialist registrar grades have been reformed into a specialty registrar (StR) grade, with more than 18,000 training places made available in this grade which will begin from August 2007.

Further information
www.mmc.nhs.uk
Modernising Medical Careers – the next steps: the future shape of foundation, specialist and general practice training programmes, UK Health Departments, April 2004.
Briefing 19: Modernising Medical Careers: a new era in medical training, NHS Employers, June 2006.

Productivity

The NHS is facing increasing pressure to improve workforce productivity. Trusts are now measured on a range of workforce productivity indicators developed by the NHS Institute. These cover:
- staff turnover
- absence levels
- use of temporary staff
- finished consultant episodes.

Finished consultant episodes are used as a measure of the amount of work undertaken by medical staff. Data on relative performance on this measure has been collected and sent to the NHS for use in local discussion on improving productivity. These measures are being kept under review.

NHS Jobs
NHS Jobs is an online recruitment service with details of job vacancies throughout the NHS in England and Wales. Launched in 2003, it has attracted more than one million registered job-seekers and more than 640 employers, and has become a key way for employers to manage recruitment more efficiently and cost-effectively. It is among the top five UK job websites, and is estimated to save the NHS £40 million a year in advertising and administration costs.

Further information
Briefing 15: NHS Jobs – key benefits for the NHS, NHS Employers, April 2006.
www.jobs.nhs.uk

Spotlight on policy: 18-week wait

One of the major workforce challenges facing the NHS is how to achieve the 18-week target from referral to treatment. The Large Scale Workforce Change Team of NHS Employers is working with trusts on how to achieve this target. Issues that are emerging include best use of administrative staff, changing roles in diagnostics and community-based staff such as community matrons.
www.18weeks.nhs.uk/public/default.aspx

Key organisation: NHS Institute for Innovation and Improvement

The Institute superseded the NHS Modernisation Agency in 2005. A special health authority based at Warwick University, it aims to promote a culture of innovation and lifelong learning for all NHS staff. It supports the rapid adoption and spread of new ideas by providing practical guidance on local, safe implementation. With an annual budget of £80 million, the NHS Institute is particularly interested in service transformation, technology and product innovation, leadership development and learning.
www.institute.nhs.uk

Pay

The wages and conditions of NHS staff are developed mainly through collective bargaining between the NHS and staff organisations, which also represent staff on a wide range of other employment issues. Most staff are members of trade unions or professional associations, and the NHS seeks 'partnership working' on key employment issues. Most NHS staff organisations have a professional and collective bargaining role. For example, the Royal College of Nursing operates as a trade union as well as a professional body, while the public service union Unison offers services on professional issues. Unison and the First Division Association have set up Managers in Partnership, an organisation to represent NHS managers' collective interests.

Although GPs are independent self-employed contractors, the contract which sets their income is negotiated by the British Medical Association, which also represents the interests of all doctors.

Agenda for Change: pay system
The Agenda for Change pay system agreed in 2004 has now largely been implemented. Almost all staff have been assimilated into the new pay structures based on a single job evaluation system, and there is now a common set of conditions of service for most NHS staff. Under Agenda for Change most staff enjoyed real pay increases and now have the opportunity for better pay progression.

One of the main aims of the system was to ensure equal pay and it is widely recognised as having achieved this objective. There are some legal challenges against the NHS arising from alleged discrimination in the pay systems before Agenda for Change. Negotiations continue for a new package of payments for unsocial hours.

The new NHS pay system is linked to the development of an NHS Knowledge and Skills Framework, which sets out the skills needed for a particular post and is linked to the job evaluation system and pay progression. Staff roles are gradually being assessed under the Knowledge and Skills Framework. This should create a 'skills escalator' which promotes education and career development.

Equal pay

Agenda for Change was designed to deliver an equal pay proof system for the NHS. The job evaluation system that underpins the new system and harmonised conditions of service should provide a defence against equal pay claims in the future. However, since the introduction of Agenda for Change, a significant number of grievances and employment tribunal claims, mostly in the north of England, have been raised against NHS organisations by trades unions and contingency fee lawyers. The NHS Litigation Authority has been given responsibility for supporting employers in the management of these claims.

Further information
www.nhsemployers.org/agendaforchange

Contract for GPs

The current GP contract for general medical services (GMS) was implemented across the UK in 2004 and revisions to the contract were introduced in April 2006, following negotiations between NHS Employers and the British Medical Association's General Practitioners Committee (GPC). The GMS contract aims to reward practices for providing high-quality care, improve GPs' working lives and ensure patients benefit from a wider range of services in the community.

The GMS contract:
- is between the PCT and the practice rather than with each GP. This is intended to give practices greater freedom to design service for local needs while encouraging better teamworking and skill mix
- helps GPs to manage their workload by enabling practices to transfer some services – including out-of-hours services – to their PCT.

A key component of the GMS contract is the Quality and Outcomes Framework (QOF), which resources and rewards practices for delivering high-quality care. The framework, which was reviewed in 2006/07, sets out a range of national standards based on the best available research evidence. The standards are divided into four domains:
- clinical standards linked to the care of patients suffering from chronic disease
- organisational standards relating to records and information, communicating with patients, education and training, medicines management and clinical and practice management
- additional services, covering cervical screening, child health surveillance, maternity services and contraceptive services
- patient experience, based on patient surveys and length of consultations.

A set of indicators has been developed for each domain to describe different aspects of performance. Practices are free to choose the domains on which they want to focus and the quality standards to which they aspire.

Further information
www.nhsemployers.org

Contract for consultants

The current consultants' contract, agreed in 2003 with amendments made in 2005, was designed to provide a more effective system of planning and timetabling consultants' duties and activities for the NHS. It gives NHS employers the ability to manage consultants' time in ways that best meet local service needs and priorities. For consultants, it means greater transparency about the commitments expected of them, along with greater clarity over the support they need from employers to make the maximum effective contribution to improving patient services.

Existing consultants were given the opportunity to take up the new contract and could choose whether or not to do so, but NHS employers no longer offer any other type of contract. Nor will they offer any other contract to newly appointed consultants.

Staff grade and associate specialists

Negotiations on a new contract for staff grade and associate specialist doctors is continuing between NHS Employers and the British Medical Association, with agreement expected during 2007.

The NHS as an employer

The NHS recognises staff as its greatest asset and knows that to recruit and retain the right people it needs to practise excellence in employment. This includes treating staff with respect and supporting them in their work; valuing equality and diversity; ensuring a healthy workplace; offering flexible working; and providing training and opportunities for development.

Sampling staff morale

The attitudes of staff are known to have an effect on the quality of patient care and can also be used to assess the performance of NHS organisations as employers. For the last three years the Healthcare Commission has measured NHS staff attitudes through the NHS staff survey. The latest survey, published in 2006, covered 209,000 staff in 570 NHS trusts in England. It showed that staff remain generally satisfied in their jobs, but overall satisfaction had declined since the 2003 survey.

Further information
NHS national staff survey 2005, Healthcare Commission, March 2006.

Equality and diversity

The NHS aims to incorporate equality and diversity into all its workforce strategies and to highlight how these can contribute to improved health and better access to health services.

Positively Diverse is the overarching programme for promoting equality and diversity in NHS organisations. The programme enables organisations to assess the extent to which NHS staff are treated fairly and equitably, regardless of their background. It also helps organisations to develop the knowledge and capacity to build, manage and retain a diverse workforce, reflecting the communities that they serve.

Further information
Age diversity in the workforce – how age profiling can benefit your organisation, NHS Employers, April 2006.
Positively Diverse: quick guide, NHS Employers, 2005.
Producing a disability equality scheme, NHS Employers, 2006.
Equality impact assessment process, NHS Employers, November 2006.

Stress and bullying

Stress is estimated to cause 30 per cent of sickness absence and cost the NHS up to £400 million a year. A campaign ran throughout 2006 to encourage employers to carry out risk assessments and change their policies and procedures to reduce stress in the workplace. It also included information to help staff spot the signs of stress and offered advice on what to do about it.

The NHS staff survey found that 15 per cent of staff felt they had been bullied or harassed by other staff. NHS Employers has developed model policy, employer and staff guidance, HR toolkits and communications materials for both employers and staff to tackle bullying.

7

Information technology in the NHS

National Programme for IT

The NHS in England is currently investing £6.2 billion in information technology over ten years. (NHSScotland has its own national eHealth IM&T strategy, see page 177; NHS Wales also has its own approach, Informing Healthcare, see page 192.) National systems will replace organisations' separate IT systems that do not communicate with each other. Once installed, the new IT infrastructure will connect more than 100,000 doctors, 380,000 nurses and 50,000 other healthcare professionals, giving patients access to their personal health and care information while transforming the way the NHS works. The National Programme for IT (NPfIT) is intended to ensure that lost records, inconvenient appointments and delayed test results become a thing of the past. The National Audit Office commented in 2006: 'The programme's scope, vision and complexity are wider and more extensive than any ongoing or planned healthcare IT programme in the world, and it represents the largest single IT investment in the UK to date'.

In addition to national IT spending, trusts are expected to increase their investment in – for example – payroll, finance and HR systems in line with the 2002 Wanless Report's recommendation that they should devote 4 per cent of their budgets to IT by 2008. Wanless (see page 113) made several key recommendations for IT in the NHS:
- doubling the IT budget and ensuring that funding is not used to subsidise other services
- stringent, centrally managed national standards for data and IT
- better management of IT implementation, including a national programme.

Wanless commented: 'Without a major advance in the effective use of ICT, the health service will find it increasingly difficult to deliver the efficient, high-quality service which the public will demand. This is a major priority which will have a crucial impact on the health service over future years.'

Implementing NPfIT does not involve a 'big bang'. Systems and services are being gradually phased in over the next few years, according to priorities and when NHS organisations are ready to implement them:
- **Phase one** Choose and Book, electronic transmission of prescriptions, and the NHS Care Records Service began during 2004/05
- **Phase two**, up to 2008, includes a richer NHS Care Records Service, with core data and reference links to local electronic patient record systems for full-record access, all patient appointments, and telemedicine starting to be established
- **Phase three** 2008–10 will provide ambulance telemonitoring in emergency response vehicles, home telemonitoring in homes requiring it, and a unified health record with social care information.

The infrastructure will include:
- the NHS Care Records Service (CRS)
- Choose and Book, the electronic booking service
- Electronic Prescriptions Service (EPS)
- a national broadband IT network (N3)
- picture archiving and communications systems (PACS)
- IT supporting GP payments, including the quality management and analysis system (QMAS)
- NHSmail, a central e-mail and directory service for the NHS
- HealthSpace and nhs.uk.

The National Audit Office (NAO) noted in 2006 that NPfIT had made 'substantial progress', but that successful implementation continued to present 'significant challenges', especially in:
- ensuring that IT suppliers deliver systems that meet the NHS's needs to agreed timescales without further slippage
- ensuring NHS organisations fully play their part in implementation
- winning the support of NHS staff and the public in making the best use of the systems to improve services.

It was not yet possible to assess NPfIT's value for money, the NAO said. Others have expressed concerns about overspending and missed timescales.

Further information
Department of Health: The National Programme for IT in the NHS, NAO, June 2006.
The NHS in England: the operating framework for 2007/08 – guidance on preparation of local IM&T plans, DH, December 2006.

Who does what
NPfIT's central team manages national procurements, oversees development of IT systems and services, and co-ordinates implementation activities. Assisting with the implementation are:
- service implementation team (SIT) – works with clinicians and other staff to ensure they can exploit the new technology's potential; SIT has seven clinical leads – representing GPs, hospital doctors, nurses and allied health professionals – to influence and improve the technologies with their own ideas
- national application service providers (NASPs) – responsible for services common to all users
- national infrastructure service provider – responsible for providing networking and support services
- clusters – each cluster comprises several strategic health authorities (SHAs) that together procure and implement NPfIT locally
- local service providers (LSPs) – each cluster has an LSP, responsible for delivering and supporting services locally. The LSP will ensure the integration of existing local systems
- SHAs, working with NHS trusts, PCTs and primary care organisations are responsible for co-ordinating mainstream investment and modernisation activities.

Key organisation: NHS Connecting for Health

NHS Connecting for Health is an agency of the Department of Health, set up in 2005. Its main role is to deliver the National Programme for IT and maintain the business systems on which the NHS relies. It is the successor body to the NHS Information Authority, and was formed as a result of the review of arm's-length bodies (see page 16). Its staff are drawn from across the NHS, civil service, academe and the private sector, and encompass management, IT, clinical and medical skills.

NHS Connecting for Health is delivering NPfIT in England only. Scotland and Wales are developing their own IT programmes, but NHS Connecting for Health recognises the importance of compatibility. The UK Information Management & Technology Forum has been set up to provide the opportunity for interaction between policy leads responsible for health informatics from England, Wales, Scotland and Northern Ireland. In addition, the Information Standards Board has representatives from each of the home countries.
 www.connectingforhealth.nhs.uk

NHS Care Records Service (CRS)

A single electronic record system to which all care providers have access is essential because patients attend various institutions at different times, encountering a range of care professionals and organisations, including social services and the independent sector. The NHS Care Records Service will connect GPs and trusts in a single, secure national system, providing all 50 million NHS patients in England with an individual electronic care record detailing key treatments in the health service or social care.

Every patient will have a two-part care record. The detailed care record will be formed from the detailed notes made by every healthcare professional who treats the patient; the summary care record will contain essential information selected from the detailed care record, such as allergies or medication.

Clinical need and patient wishes will decide who has access to records. Access to the computer system will only be allowed after training, and users must register to obtain an NHS 'smart card' with a chip and personal identification number. Users must be directly involved in the care of the patient whose record they wish to access, and access will depend on their role: for example, a receptionist booking an appointment will only have access to basic information to identify a patient and make the booking. Every time someone accesses a patient's record, a note will be made of who, when and what they did. Patients can request this information. The CRS Registration Authority is responsible for registering and verifying the identity of NHS staff who need to access records. By 2008, people will have private and secure access to a summary version of their own record whenever they want, using HealthSpace (see page 44).

A core data storage and messaging system, known as 'the Spine', is central to the CRS. In addition to storing patients' personal characteristics, summarised clinical information and security systems, this will offer a secondary users' service, providing anonymised data for business reports and statistics for research and planning.

The first phase of implementation was completed during 2004, and included the infrastructure to enable booking of outpatient appointments and professionals to view basic patient information. A PCT 'early adopter' programme to implement the summary care record began in 2007. Full implementation should be completed by 2010.

In addition, the GP2GP record transfer project is piloting the electronic transfer of patients' healthcare records from one GP surgery to another. By March 2007, 500 practices were using the system, which is designed to ensure records are available to the new GP within 24 hours of a patient registering with their practice.

www.nhscarerecords.nhs.uk

Choose and Book

Choose and Book, the electronic booking service, is designed to underpin the Government's policy of enabling patients to choose which hospital to attend at a date and time to suit them. The software allows GPs and other primary care staff to make initial hospital or clinic outpatient appointments before the patient has left the surgery. This will enable clinicians to track referrals more easily and conduct e-mail discussion about cases when necessary. It will also provide more consistent, accurate and efficient referral information without the delays of paper correspondence. Choose and Book should reduce the chance of patients not turning up for appointments and improve clinical governance by providing an audit trail.

By the end of 2006, 85 per cent of GP practices were using Choose and Book, representing 28 per cent of NHS referral activity from GP surgery to specialist care. It has made more than one million bookings since its introduction in 2004. When fully operational, the system is expected to take 190,000 bookings a week.

www.chooseandbook.nhs.uk

Electronic prescription service

The Electronic Transmission of Prescriptions programme will create and implement the electronic prescription service (EPS), then integrate it with the NHS CRS. EPS will operate throughout England.

With electronic transmission, prescriptions are transferred electronically to the pharmacist nominated by the patient. If a pharmacy has not been nominated, the patient is given an ePrescription to present at a pharmacy. This has a barcode which enables the community pharmacist to obtain details of the prescription from the NHS CRS. The prescribed medication details are added to the patient's electronic record held by the NHS CRS. Electronic transmission will increase patient safety by reducing prescription errors and providing better information at the point of prescribing and dispensing. This also creates the opportunity to reduce adverse drug events where the patient responds poorly to medication. By the beginning of 2007, more than 10 million electronic prescription messages had been transmitted using EPS, and the first stage of the service was live in 24 per cent of GP surgeries and 36 per cent of community pharmacies. In due course, other locations such as walk-in centres and dental practices will be included. There are also plans to include hospitals.

N3: the New National Network

N3 is replacing the private NHS communications network, NHSnet. It will link all NHS locations in England electronically for the first time. N3 promises sufficient connectivity and broadband capacity to meet the NHS's current and future needs, and will provide the essential technical infrastructure for NPfIT's other major projects. Among its benefits, clinicians will be able to send high-quality images to specialists for remote diagnosis and use it for secure clinical messaging. It should also make video conferencing and remote working much easier.

Connections to the new N3 network started in April 2004. Implementation is expected to take about three years to complete. More than 15,500 connections had been made by late 2006, including 97 per cent of GP surgeries. More than 830,000 NHS employees were able to make use of N3.

NHSmail
NHSmail is a secure national e-mail and directory service for NHS staff, developed specifically to meet the British Medical Association's requirements for clinical e-mail between NHS organisations. It provides a national directory of people in the NHS, containing the name, e-mail addresses, telephone numbers, name and address of their NHS organisation, and information about departments, job roles and specialties. Staff are assigned an e-mail address that moves with them if they change their job or location within the NHS.

Further information
A guide to the national programme for information technology, NHS Connecting for Health, 2005.

The electronic NHS

NHSweb
Websites can be hosted exclusively on NHSnet for NHS use, and are described as being on NHSweb as opposed to being on the worldwide web. NHSweb also hosts intranets for individual NHS organisations. Users connected to other networks are blocked at the firewall and cannot access NHSweb sites, although they may send e-mails.

nhs.uk
This is the official gateway to NHS organisations on the internet. It provides staff and the public with information about the NHS at a local and national level, including directories of all NHS organisations and the services they offer.
www.nhs.uk

NHS number

The NHS number is the common currency of NHS information and fundamental to NPfIT. It is a unique identifier that provides a common link between a patient's records – both electronic and manual – across the NHS. It consists of ten digits: the first nine are the identifier and the tenth is a check digit used to confirm the number's validity. It is the cornerstone of the move towards an electronic health record, and enables disparate information to be collated to build a comprehensive record of a person's health.

One significant drawback in achieving full use of the NHS number was that babies were not issued with it until their birth was registered. This resulted in delays up to six weeks, during which time they might undergo complex treatment spanning several organisations.

NHS Numbers For Babies (NN4B) was launched in 2002, which means that all patients, including babies, now have an NHS number from birth for life. NHS numbers are put on any documentation related to the baby such as the antenatal record, the parent-held child health record and the hospital's discharge summary.

National Library for Health (NLH)

The National Library for Health is a comprehensive web resource that brings together all NHS library and information services. It aims to collect in one place trusted, authoritative information resources, providing seamless access to the best available evidence wherever, and whenever, it is needed. Its services include:
- specialist libraries – web-based collections containing clinical and non-clinical information on major health priority areas
- clinical information and summaries of evidence
- bibliographic databases and contents tables to support research
- collections of full-text e-journals and e-books
- a comprehensive search engine
- current awareness services
- clinical question answering
- a range of national and local services provided by library staff.

Further information

Briefing 110: National Library for Health Management, NHS Confederation, November 2004.
www.library.nhs.uk

Information Centre for Health and Social Care

The Information Centre for Health and Social Care aims to co-ordinate and streamline the collection and sharing of data about health and adult social care. Set up in 2005, its remit is to be 'a focus for everyone who needs information, including patients, clinicians and regulators'. It is attempting to simplify and streamline data collection processes, and reduce the time spent annually on data collections in the NHS to 400 people years.

Further information
Information Centre for Health and Social Care: www.ic.nhs.uk
Briefing 120: Reducing the burden of data collection – the NHS Health and Social Care Information Centre, NHS Confederation, July 2005.

PRIMIS +

PRIMIS+ (formerly Primary Care Information Services) provides training and assistance to information and data-quality facilitators employed by PCTs or local health informatics services. These facilitators then 'cascade' their knowledge and skills to local GPs and practice staff. PRIMIS+ is managed by NHS Connecting for Health and based at Nottingham University's division of primary care.
www.primis.nhs.uk

THE NHS CONFEDERATION   NHS Employers

Put these dates in your diary...

NHS Confederation annual conference and exhibition
18 – 20 June 2008
Manchester
www.nhsconfed.org

NHS Employers annual conference and exhibition
4 – 6 November 2008
Birmingham
www.nhsemployers.org

8
Public sector partnerships

The concept of partnership has become a cornerstone of policy for modernising institutions across the whole field of civil and public life. It is one of the NHS's ten core principles, and new partnership arrangements – with local government, the voluntary and private sectors and indeed with patients and the public – are a central feature of health and social care policy. Partnership is no longer an add-on but a fundamental characteristic of public sector modernisation, and evidence is increasing that good partnership working improves services.

The practical benefits of partnership working include:
- developing commissioning through co-operation rather than competitive tendering, so getting the best from all local groups instead of limiting choice and creating local tensions
- providing joint training to foster understanding of wider local issues and others' ways of working
- helping join up the health and government agenda on strategic planning, aligning local delivery plans with local authorities' community planning processes
- setting a framework for pooling budgets, providing joint services and developing joint strategic approaches to community involvement
- enabling joint data-gathering and developing common indicators and targets.

Further information
Getting closer: a guide to partnerships in new health policy, NHS Confederation, 2002.

Local authorities

The Government's priorities and planning framework treats the health and social care system as one, with shared-lead priorities where both health and social care organisations have a major contribution to make. Wales's 22 local health boards are coterminous with unitary local authorities. In Northern Ireland the NHS has been responsible for both health and social care since 1972, and its proposed local commissioning groups will be coterminous with seven new district councils. In Scotland, community health partnerships have increased coterminosity between NHS and local authority boundaries.

In all areas, joint working and the engagement of local authorities are required – especially in tackling health inequalities, expanding intermediate care, implementing national service frameworks, improving services for vulnerable people and those with long-term conditions, as well as tackling neighbourhood renewal.

The white paper, *Our health, our care, our say*, noted that, 'People do not care about organisational boundaries when seeking support or help, and expect services to reflect this'. The Government is keen to see more co-location of health and social care services, a principle endorsed in the consultation that preceded the white paper. Community hospitals may offer one way of doing this, and the Government has promised to support the NHS and local government 'in developing more effective partnerships to fund and develop joint capital projects'. Other measures include:
- further development of local area agreements to strengthen partnerships
- integration of health and social care planning cycles
- joint health and social care plans for people with long-term conditions
- a single complaints procedure across health and social care
- a national framework for NHS continuing care assessments
- further guidance on the director of adult social services' role, with emphasis on working in local health and social care partnerships
- strengthening the public health director's role to link it more closely with overview and scrutiny committees (see page 146)
- national criteria on means testing services and a commitment to extend personalised budgets and direct payments.

The local government white paper, *Strong and prosperous communities*, reinforced partnership working and will have a particular impact on PCTs – especially by making it easier for them to work with local authorities to tackle health inequalities. Upper-tier local authorities will have a duty to prepare local area agreements (see page 146) in consultation with PCTs, NHS trusts and foundation trusts.

New statutory partnerships for health and well-being will be created, with responsibilities likely to include:
- agreement of shared outcomes
- a common assessment framework
- single budgets where appropriate
- joint commissioning and planning
- delivery of joint local area agreement targets
- a consistent approach to patient and public involvement
- support for high-quality personalised provision, including capacity in the third sector.

Further information
Strong and prosperous communities. The local government white paper, Communities and Local Government, October 2006.
Briefing 139: The local government white paper proposals, NHS Confederation, November 2006.

Encouraging co-operation through legislation
New powers to enable health and local authority partners to work together more effectively were contained in Section 31 of the 1999 Health Act and came into force in 2000. The Local Government and Public Involvement in Health Bill 2006 will extend the duty of the NHS and local authorities to co-operate – as outlined in the local government white paper (see above) – when it becomes law.

The Health Act created a duty of co-operation between NHS bodies and local authorities in England and Wales. It provides for them to develop together local strategies for improving health and healthcare, and allows them to make joint arrangements for purchasing or providing health and health-related services – for example, social care. Strategic health authorities, primary care trusts, social services, housing, transport, leisure and library services, community and many acute services can all be involved.

Specifically, the Act introduced flexibilities to enable NHS organisations and local authorities to set up:
- pooled funds – to be spent on agreed projects for designated services
- lead commissioning – they can agree to delegate commissioning of a service to one lead organisation
- integrated provision – combining staff, resources and management structures to integrate a service from managerial level to the front line.

PCTs have the key role in representing the NHS in developing partnerships. For this they are required to work flexibly, particularly with local authorities, which may operate on a different geography from individual PCTs. This means that in practice a network of PCTs may have to work collaboratively with an organisation or partnership.

The NHS and local government have clear, common aims, objectives and activity, much of which contributes to delivering NHS priorities. Involvement in planning, prioritising and delivering strategic planning provides ways of engaging with local communities and the voluntary sector and ensures stakeholders' involvement in NHS planning objectives.

The Children Act 2004 enhances the NHS's role in working with local partners to safeguard children. For example, NHS trusts and local authorities can pool their children's budgets. The Act set up the role of children's commissioner for England and established a statutory duty for all agencies working with children to co-operate.

The Local Government and Public Involvement in Health Bill will:
- create local involvement networks (LINks – see page 66) – local authorities will have a duty to make contractual arrangements to involve people in commissioning, provision and scrutiny of health and social services
- strengthen and clarify requirements for public involvement and consultation on the provision of health services
- introduce a duty on each PCT to report on consultation arrangements.

Further information
Communities and Local Government www.communities.gov.uk
Department for Education and Skills www.dfes.gov.uk/childrenandfamilies

Spotlight on policy: local area agreements

Local area agreements (LAAs) aim to improve local public services by providing a new framework for the relationship between central and local government. They cover one or more local authorities, and focus on a collection of goals across a range of services that relate to either national or local priorities. To set these priorities the local authority liaises with other organisations, which pool or align their budgets in order to achieve them. The Government Office for the Region handles the negotiations with the local authority and its partners, with regional public health directors representing health interests.

The LAA is then sent to ministers for approval. Proposed LAAs are sent to the Secretary of State for Health accompanied by the regional public health director's assessment of the health content and a view as to whether the LAA should be agreed. LAAs are structured around four key themes:
- children and young people
- safer and stronger communities
- health and older people.
- economic development.

Further information
Background briefing 1: Local public service agreements, NHS Confederation, June 2005.

Overview and scrutiny committees (OSCs)
The Health and Social Care Act 2001 gave local authorities specific powers to scrutinise local health services and health organisations. These powers formally rest with authorities that have social services responsibilities (county, unitary, metropolitan, London borough authorities), but there are provisions for joint or delegated scrutiny with borough or district councils.

OSCs are made up of elected council members not on the authority's executive or cabinet. They are able to call chief executives of local health organisations to attend a scrutiny hearing at least twice a year. But overview and scrutiny should be more than twice-yearly adversarial confrontations, giving an opportunity to build

on existing partnership arrangements and examine services across health and local authorities. OSCs can:
- refer contested service changes to the Secretary of State
- report their recommendations locally
- insist on being consulted by the NHS over major changes to health services.

The Centre for Public Scrutiny helped to foster local authorities' role in scrutinising health services by running a support programme. It has published a guide for health OSCs, clarifying their distinct roles.

Further information
Centre for Public Scrutiny: **www.cfps.org.uk**
Local authority health overview and scrutiny committees & patient and public involvement forums: working together – a practical guide, CfPS, July 2005.
A guide to the NHS for members and officers of health scrutiny committees, DH, November 2003.

Integrated Care Network
The Integrated Care Network is an initiative run by the DH in partnership with the NHS Confederation, Local Government Association and others. Its purpose is to:
- lead and co-ordinate development of integrated working
- support frontline agencies working to integrate services
- increase use of the Health Act flexibilities, children's trust and care trust facilities
- support those responsible for ensuring frontline agencies deliver their objectives
- contribute to policy development
- join up working with other stakeholders, governmental and non-governmental
- maximise funding opportunities.

Further information
www.integratedcarenetwork.gov.uk
Integration and partnership working: what's working, not working and how it can be encouraged, ICN, December 2005.

Spotlight on policy: reimbursement for delayed discharge

Better joint working between health and social care has reduced the number of mainly older people occupying acute hospital beds even though they are ready to be discharged. Many delays were due to social services departments being slow to assess the patient for community services or because they could not provide the services the patient needed on leaving hospital.

Under the Community Care (Delayed Discharges) Act 2003, local authorities must reimburse NHS acute trusts if social care assessments and social services are the sole reason for delaying discharge. Some patients' discharges are delayed due to lack of NHS services. Proper assessment on admission indicates whether someone is likely to need social services on leaving hospital. Hospitals must ensure that internal processes, such as pharmacy and patient transport, can contribute to the discharge plan within this timescale.

These arrangements were introduced in 2004, and cover acute inpatient delayed discharges only. Figures show delayed discharges fell from over 6 per cent of patients in 2001/02 to 2.1 per cent in 2005/06. Since 2006, general non-acute and mental health trusts have been tackling delayed discharges. At mid-year, about 10 per cent of patients in general non-acute beds and 9 per cent of patients in mental health beds were experiencing delayed discharge.

Further information
The Community Care (Delayed Discharges Etc) Act 2003: guidance for implementation (HSC 2003/009), DH, September 2003.
Learning materials for effective hospital discharge:
www.dischargetraining.doh.gov.uk

Other partnerships

Local strategic partnerships (LSPs)
LSPs are intended to:
- bring together the different parts of the public sector and the private, business, community and voluntary sectors
- enable strategic decisions to be taken while still being close enough to individual neighbourhoods to allow decisions to be made at community level
- create strengthened, empowered, healthier and safer communities.

The NHS has a key role to play in LSPs and neighbourhood renewal by providing improving health and reducing health inequalities.

The core tasks of LSPs are to:
- develop and deliver a local neighbourhood renewal strategy to secure more jobs, better education, improved health, reduced crime and better housing, narrowing the gap between deprived neighbourhoods and the rest and contributing to the national targets to tackle deprivation
- prepare and implement a community strategy for the area, identify and deliver the most important things that need to be done, keep track of progress and keep it up to date
- bring together local plans, partnerships and initiatives to provide a forum through which mainstream service providers (local authorities, police, health services, central government agencies and bodies outside the public sector) work effectively together to meet local needs and priorities
- work with local authorities that are developing a local public service agreement to help devise and meet suitable targets.

Voluntary organisations: the Compact
The Compact is an agreement between the Government and the voluntary and community sector, made in 1998. It is designed to improve their relationship for mutual advantage, with commitments on both sides. It is based on principles – such as recognising groups are independent and have the right to campaign – which have been turned into codes of practice on funding, consultation and volunteering. The national Compact ensures that voluntary and community activity is supported and encouraged, and includes black and minority ethnic groups. In 2006 the Government appointed a commissioner for the Compact, whose role is to champion its full implementation at every level.

Local compacts are similar agreements but at local level with councils and other public bodies. One-third of local authority areas are covered by a local compact.

Community and voluntary groups play important health roles: they support service users, act as advocates or lobbyists, provide a range of health services and are a conduit for information, particularly on health promotion. Local community groups with an interest or role in health or social care are vital sources of expertise on specialist areas.

All NHS organisations in England should now be signed up to a local compact.

A strategic agreement in 2004 between the DH, the NHS and the voluntary sector aimed to make it easier for the sector to provide services for the NHS. The agreement is designed to complement the Compact. A national strategic partnership forum is responsible for reviewing how the agreement is working, supporting local partnerships in lowering barriers between the NHS and the voluntary sector and pulling together best practice and innovation.

Voluntary and independent sector providers of NHS and social services are now eligible for affiliate membership of the NHS Confederation.
www.thecompact.org.uk

Government departments
A range of Government departments – apart from the DH – have responsibilities that impinge on health, and work in partnership with the NHS. They include:

Communities and Local Government
Responsible for housing, regional and local government, as well as overseeing the Social Exclusion Unit, the Neighbourhood Renewal Unit and the Government Offices for the Regions.
www.communities.gov.uk

Home Office
Lead responsibility for progress on the drug strategy; the Home Secretary chairs the cross-government Cabinet ministerial sub-committee on drugs policy.; local crime and disorder reduction partnerships.
www.homeoffice.gov.uk/drugs
www.drugs.gov.uk

Department for Education and Skills
Responsible for children's social care policy, the Change for Children programme, Every Child Matters strategy and Sure Start, which aims to improve health, education and emotional development for young children in disadvantaged areas. The Healthy Schools programme is run jointly with the DH.
www.surestart.gov.uk
www.dfes.gov.uk

Department for Environment, Food and Rural Affairs
Responsibilities include water, farming, fisheries, horticulture and some aspects of rural health and well-being. Protection from the effects of pollution or toxic chemicals are particular concerns.
www.defra.gov.uk

Prison healthcare
Since April 2006, primary care trusts have been responsible for commissioning healthcare for prisons. The aim is to provide prisoners with access to the same quality and range of healthcare services as the public receives from the NHS.

A national partnership agreement between the DH and the Home Office on behalf of the Prison Service underpins the local partnership arrangements between PCTs and public sector prisons.

Further information
National partnership agreement between the Department of Health and the Home Office for the accountability and commissioning of health services for prisoners in public sector prisons in England, DH, January 2007.

Public health

Public health is concerned with improving the population's health, rather than treating the diseases of individual patients. The official definition of public health, devised by former Chief Medical Officer Sir Donald Acheson, is: 'the science and art of preventing disease, prolonging life, and promoting health through the organised efforts of society'. Many of the aims of public health can only be achieved through partnerships across Government departments and between the Government, NHS, local authorities, and the private and voluntary sectors.

> **Key text:** *Health, work and well-being*

This is a joint strategy document in a 'groundbreaking partnership' from the DH, Department for Work and Pensions and the Health and Safety Executive about improving the health of working-age people. Its aim is 'to break the link between ill health and inactivity, to advance the prevention of ill health and injury, to encourage good management of occupational health, and to transform opportunities for people to recover from illness while at work'.

Health, work and well-being – caring for our future: a strategy for the health and well-being of working age people, DWP, DH & HSE, October 2005.

Further information
Inside Track leading edge briefing: Incapacity benefit reform and the NHS, NHS Confederation, October 2005. In keeping with the Government's successful Pathways to Work project, this examines the role the NHS has to play in the reform of incapacity benefit. It explores the challenges facing health organisations and clinicians in supporting people to retain and regain employment following physical and mental ill health.

Public health professionals monitor the health status of the community, identify health needs, develop programmes to reduce risk and screen for early disease, control communicable disease, promote health, plan and evaluate healthcare provision and manage and implement change.

Choosing health – the public health white paper
Choosing health is based on the principle that the NHS should improve health and prevent disease, not just provide treatment for those who are ill. The white paper encompasses the Government's view that people should make their own choices about their lifestyle, and consequently their health, but that these should be informed by good information and advice about the choices available. The NHS will help, support and encourage people to choose healthy lifestyles.

Principles behind the new approach to public health are:
- informed choices – people want to be able to make their own decisions about choices that affect their health and to have good-quality information to help them do so
- personalisation – support has to be tailored to the realities of individual lives
- working together – progress depends on effective partnerships across communities.

Measures covered in the white paper include:
- a ban on smoking in the workplace; restaurants serving alcohol and pubs preparing food must ban smoking unless they apply for a special licence
- an overhaul of sexual health services
- action to safeguard children's health, including curbs on the promotion of unhealthy foods to children
- clear, unambiguous labelling of the nutritional content of food
- NHS health trainers to provide advice to individuals on how to improve their lifestyles
- specialist obesity services within every PCT.

The public health white paper is a landmark document that promotes a genuine cross-governmental approach to public health, pushing it towards the top of priorities across the whole spectrum of government. It recognises the significant health benefits that could be gained by tackling public health issues, and it acknowledges – importantly – that the NHS cannot solve all health-related problems on its own.

Two years after the white paper's publication, the DH issued an update on progress in *Health Challenge England*. It found:
- life expectancy increasing across the board
- housing-stock quality improved
- more children lifted out of poverty
- mortality rates for cancer and circulatory diseases for people under 75 have fallen annually since the mid-1990s
- 1.2 million fewer people smoking than in 1998
- the gap between the most disadvantaged areas and the national average narrowed
- a consistent north–south divide, with people in the north of England experiencing poorer health than those in the south
- life expectancy one year shorter for women and two years shorter for men in the north compared to the south.

Further information
Choosing health: making healthier choices easier, DH, November 2004.
Briefing 111: the public health white paper, NHS Confederation, November 2004.
Delivering choosing health: making healthier choices easier, DH, March 2005.
Health Challenge England – next steps for choosing health, DH, October 2006.

Public health workforce
The public health workforce comprises people in a range of disciplines who work in one of three categories:
- health improvement and reducing inequalities: teachers, local business leaders, managers, social workers, transport engineers, housing officers, other local government staff and the voluntary sector, as well as doctors, nurses and other healthcare professionals
- public health practice: health visitors, environmental health officers and community development workers, and those who use research, information, public health science or health promotion skills in specific public health fields
- public health consultants and specialists, who work at a strategic or senior management level or at a senior level of scientific expertise.

Spotlight on policy: the smoking ban

Smoking in enclosed public places will be banned in England from July 2007, and has been banned in Wales and Northern Ireland since April 2007 and in Scotland since March 2006. Initial plans for a partial ban in England were scrapped as impractical and offering insufficient protection from passive smoking in places such as bars and clubs.

Anyone smoking in an enclosed public place could be fined £50, while those in charge of the premises could be fined £2,500. Failure to display no-smoking signs could lead to a £200 on-the-spot fine.

Between 1998 and 2004, the proportion of adult smokers in England fell from 28 to 25 per cent – a reduction of 1.2 million. But smoking still causes 106,000 deaths a year in the UK.

The ban follows similar decisions in other parts of Europe – the Irish Republic introduced a ban in 2004 – and the USA.

Key text: *Securing good health for the whole population* (the Wanless Report on public health)

Following Derek Wanless's 2002 report on future NHS resources (see page 113), the Government asked him to look at ill-health prevention and wider determinants of health in England, and at the cost-effectiveness of action to improve the whole population's health and reduce health inequalities.

His subsequent report, published by the Treasury in 2004, argued that urgent and concerted action was needed at all levels to shift from 'a national sickness service which treats disease to a national health service which focuses on preventing it'. Random target-setting had failed to produce results, while the Government's hopes for combating obesity were unrealistic and its goals for reducing smoking unambitious, he said.

The Government should aim for California's smoking targets, and action should be taken to reduce salt in the diet, increase exercise and screen those at high risk of diabetes. The onus was on individuals to help themselves, but much more information was needed. Wanless called for a strategy led by the Government but implemented by local authorities, primary care trusts and other local organisations.
www.hm-treasury.gov.uk

The public health system in England has ten core functions:
- health surveillance, monitoring and analysis
- investigation of disease outbreaks, epidemics and health risks
- establishing, designing and managing health promotion and disease prevention programmes
- enabling communities and citizens to promote health and reduce inequalities
- creating and sustaining cross-governmental and inter-sectoral partnerships to improve health and reduce inequalities
- ensuring compliance with regulations and laws to protect and promote health
- developing and maintaining a well-educated and trained, multidisciplinary public health workforce
- ensuring the effective performance of NHS services to meet goals in improving health, preventing disease and reducing inequalities

- research, development, evaluation and innovation
- quality-assuring the public health function.

Public Health electronic Library (PHeL): **www.phel.gov.uk**

Reducing health inequalities

This is a priority for Government because health inequalities are seen as avoidable and fundamentally unfair. Unemployment and poor housing, in particular, are major causes of ill-health. Action to break the cycle of deprivation and its impact on health is central to much Government policy. Tackling health inequalities and improving health require active commitment by Government departments and groups at all levels – national, regional and local. Joint working, partnerships, networking, shared funding and resources are crucial.

The Department of Health, with the support of 11 other Government departments, published in 2003 a three-year programme of action to carry forward the recommendations in the cross-cutting review on health inequalities in the 2002 comprehensive spending review. *Tackling health inequalities – a programme for action* covers a range of local, regional and national organisations including the NHS, local authorities, social services, education, planning and employment.

Key organisation: Health Protection Agency

The Health Protection Agency advises the Government on public health protection policies and programmes. It also supports the NHS and other agencies in protecting people from infectious diseases, poisons and chemical and radiological hazards. It provides a rapid response to health protection emergencies, including the deliberate release of biological, chemical, poisonous or radioactive substances. It merged with the National Radiological Protection Board in 2005 to form a UK-wide comprehensive health protection service. It has 300 staff. **www.hpa.org.uk**

Health inequalities programme for action: themes and principles

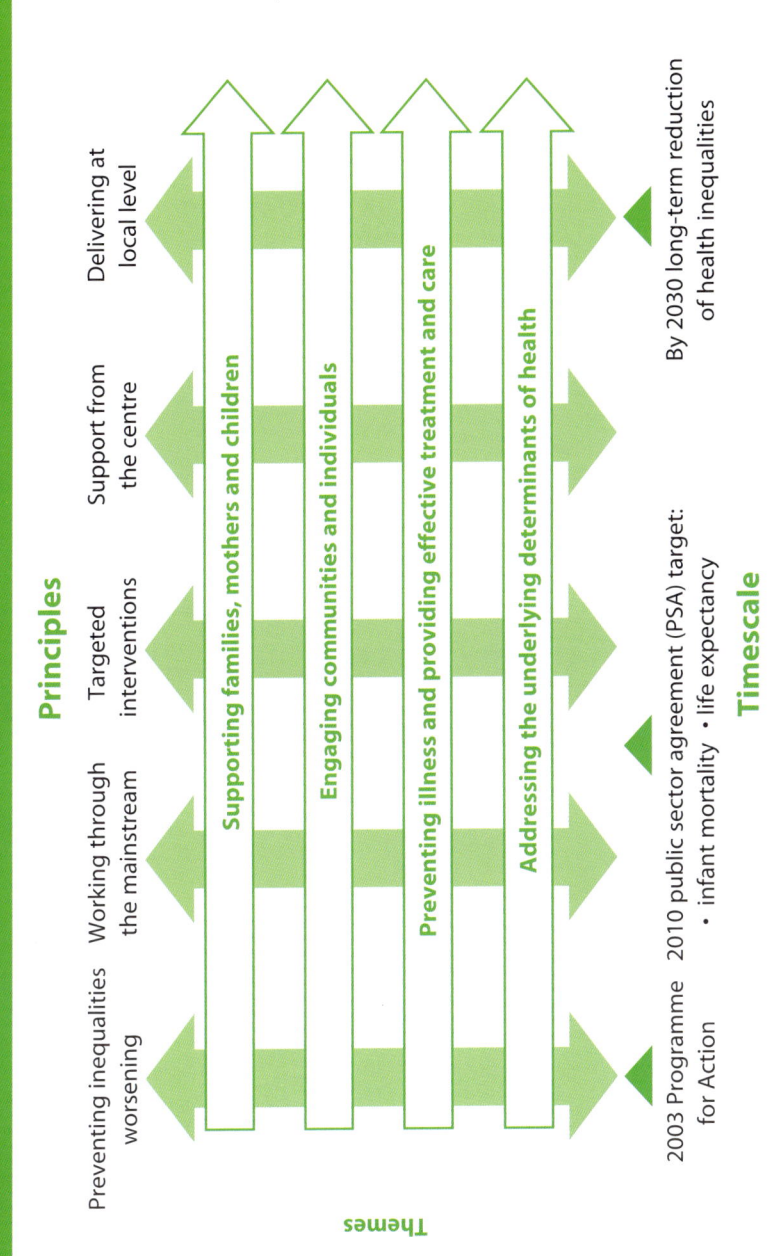

Principles

- Preventing inequalities worsening
- Working through the mainstream
- Targeted interventions
- Support from the centre
- Delivering at local level

Themes

- Supporting families, mothers and children
- Engaging communities and individuals
- Preventing illness and providing effective treatment and care
- Addressing the underlying determinants of health

Timescale

- 2003 Programme for Action
- 2010 public sector agreement (PSA) target:
  • infant mortality • life expectancy
- By 2030 long-term reduction of health inequalities

Source: *Tackling health inequalities*, Department of Health 2003

> **Key text:** *Getting ahead of the curve: a strategy for combating infectious diseases*

This sets out an infectious diseases strategy for England and was published by the DH in 2002. The strategy describes the scope and nature of the threat posed by infectious diseases, and establishes priorities for action to combat present as well as possible future threats. Among these measures are a local health protection service, a strengthened and expanded system of surveillance, rationalisation of microbiology laboratories, a programme of new vaccine development and plans to combat the deliberate release of biological, chemical or radiological agents.

Its four main themes are:
- supporting families, mothers and children to ensure the best possible start in life and break the intergenerational cycle of ill-health
- engaging communities and individuals to ensure relevance, responsiveness and sustainability
- preventing illness and providing effective treatment and care by making certain the NHS provides leadership and contributes to reducing inequalities
- addressing the underlying determinants of health by dealing with the long-term causes of health inequalities.

The programme promotes the idea that organisations, staff and individuals themselves have a role to play in tackling health inequalities. It highlights three key roles for the NHS:
- leading and supporting partnerships
- ensuring that service modernisation reduces health inequalities
- contributing to the local regeneration agenda.

PCTs are responsible locally for leading partnerships and influencing partners so that their services help improve health and reduce health inequalities.

The DH's 2004 public service agreement further raised the profile of tackling inequalities. It contains a target to reduce inequalities in health outcomes by 10 per cent by 2010, as measured by infant mortality and life expectancy at birth. The life-expectancy element focuses on reducing the health gap between the fifth of local authority areas with the lowest life expectancy at birth and the rest of the population. The infant mortality aspect of the target seeks to reduce the gap between manual groups and the rest of the population. A progress report in 2006 found slight improvements in the trends in inequalities in road accident casualties for children, educational attainment and housing quality. However, it found signs that between 2000 and 2005 inequalities in smoking in pregnancy were widening between the routine and manual group and all mothers.

A group of 'spearhead' PCTs covering 70 local authorities identified as the most health-deprived areas are piloting initiatives, such as health trainers and enhanced smoking-cessation services, to reduce health inequalities. Over a quarter of the population of England will be included in the initiative.

The NHS at national level has also appointed a director for equality and human rights 'to tackle inequalities in all aspects of health and social care delivery'.

Further information
Tackling health inequalities – a programme for action, DH, July 2003.
Briefing 90: Tackling health inequalities – a programme for action, NHS Confederation, October 2003.
Tackling health inequalities: status report on the programme for action – 2006 update of headline indicators, DH, December 2006.
Tackling health inequalities: the spearhead group of local authorities and primary care trusts, DH, November 2004.

Healthcare for asylum seekers and refugees
People with an outstanding application for refuge in the UK are entitled to use NHS services without charge. Asylum seekers are often from very different cultures, may not understand the principles behind the NHS, may not speak English and may have complex healthcare requirements.

The DH's Asylum Seeker Co-ordination Team (ASCT) co-ordinates healthcare policy for asylum seekers and refugees. ASCT works across the DH and other Government departments, and with health workers and service planners in the field. In particular, it liaises with the Home Office to try to ensure that health and social care needs are met at all stages of the asylum process and taken into account in policy planning.

Asylum seekers usually stay in a network of induction centres on their arrival. Here they undergo an initial health assessment, normally by a nurse with access to a GP. Each asylum seeker is issued with a national hand-held health record.

The best model of healthcare for asylum seekers is integration into existing mainstream services. Where this is not possible straight away, the NHS locally may have to consider dedicated initiatives appropriate for asylum seekers new to an area. Some PCTs ensure that there is space on GMS surgery lists for asylum-seekers; others use personal medical services to set up surgeries for local vulnerable populations, which may include asylum seekers. PCTs and local councils are responsible for ensuring adequate access to interpreters for asylum seekers within their own area.

Further information
Unheard voices – listening to the views of asylum-seekers and refugees, Commission for Patient and Public Involvement in Health, May 2006.
Caring for dispersed asylum seekers: a resource pack, DH, June 2003.

Government Offices for the Regions
When strategic health authorities were reorganised in 2006, their public health teams were combined with the DH's regional public health teams, which have been located in the nine Government Offices for the Regions (GOs) since 2002.

The public health teams are charged with:
- developing a cross-government and cross-sector approach to tackling the wider determinants of health
- informing regional work on economic regeneration, education, employment and transport
- ensuring there is a proper health contribution to local strategic partnerships
- accountability for the protection of health (including against communicable diseases and environmental hazards) across the region
- making sure the public health function is properly managed at local level
- emergency and disaster planning and management
- being the main point of contact for serious concerns about clinical standards and associated enquiries.

The nine GOs are: North East, North West, Yorkshire and the Humber, East Midlands, West Midlands, East of England, London, South East and South West.

Public health observatories

Public health observatories (PHOs) are closely linked to the regional public health groups. Their job is to support local bodies by:
- monitoring health and disease trends, highlighting areas for action
- identifying gaps in health information
- advising on methods for assessing the impact of health inequalities
- drawing together information from different sources in new ways to improve health
- carrying out projects to highlight particular health issues
- evaluating progress by local agencies in improving health and reducing inequality
- looking ahead to give early warning of public health problems.

The observatories are co-ordinated by the Association for Public Health Observatories. In addition, there is a Scottish PHO, the Wales Centre for Health and an Ireland and Northern Ireland PHO.

www.apho.org.uk

Healthy living centres (HLCs)

The Healthy Living Centre initiative was launched in 1999 by the Big Lottery Fund with a UK-wide budget of £300 million from lottery funds: 349 HLCs were set up before the funding deadline was reached in 2002.

The programme targets the most disadvantaged areas and groups. HLCs are expected to influence social exclusion, poor access to services and the social and economic aspects of deprivation that can contribute to health inequalities. They are expected to be accessible to 20 per cent of the population. HLCs may not be a single centre: some are programmes of activities based in existing premises, or services funded through mobile or outreach facilities. Local communities and users are expected to be involved in all aspects of a project.

Examples of projects include smoking cessation, dietary advice, physical activity, health screening programmes, training and skills schemes, arts programmes and complementary therapy.

Further information

Healthy Living Centres: year four evaluation, Big Lottery Fund, August 2006.
www.biglotteryfund.org.uk

9

The NHS in Scotland

The structure of NHSScotland

The Scottish Parliament
The Scottish Parliament opened in 1999 with powers devolved from the UK Parliament covering matters that include health, social work, education, housing and local government. Its 129 members (MSPs) can therefore pass primary and secondary legislation affecting Scotland on a range of domestic issues. Issues concerning Scotland that have a UK or international impact are dealt with by the UK Parliament. These 'reserved matters' include foreign affairs and defence, but also certain health-related issues:
- professional regulation
- abortion
- human fertilisation
- genetics
- control and safety of medicines.

The UK Parliament can also make laws that will apply to Scotland on any subject, but does not normally legislate on devolved matters without the consent of the Scottish Parliament.

Committees play a central part in the Parliament's work, taking evidence from witnesses, scrutinising legislation and conducting inquiries. The Health Committee considers health policy and matters such as community care services, public health initiatives and food safety standards. It is responsible for considering any proposed legislation which falls within its remit. This includes legislation setting out the Scottish Executive's budget proposals for each financial year. The committee also commissions research, conducts inquiries and considers petitions submitted by the public. It has nine members, assigned between the parties on a proportional basis.

In addition, some of the Parliament's eight mandatory committees take an interest in NHSScotland: for example, the Finance Committee is concerned with public expenditure and how the Scottish Executive's budget is spent, while the Audit Committee holds NHS boards to account for how they spend taxpayers' money and ensures public funds are spent effectively.

The Scotland Office, led by the Secretary of State for Scotland, represents Scottish interests in the UK Government and Parliament.

www.scottish.parliament.uk
www.scotlandoffice.gov.uk

The Scottish Executive
The Scottish Executive is the devolved government in Scotland. Its relationship with the Scottish Parliament is similar to the relationship between the UK Government and the UK Parliament at Westminster. Members of the Scottish Executive are chosen from the party or parties holding a majority of seats in the Parliament. The last elections to the Parliament were held in May 2007.

The Executive is led by a First Minister, elected by the Scottish Parliament, who appoints a cabinet of Scottish ministers. Executive civil servants are accountable to these ministers, who are themselves accountable to the Scottish Parliament. The Executive administers an annual budget of about £30 billion.

www.scotland.gov.uk

Scottish Executive Health Department (SEHD)

SEHD is responsible for NHSScotland as well as for developing and implementing health and community care policy. It provides the statutory and financial framework for NHSScotland and holds it to account for its performance. The Executive has discretion to intervene if serious problems arise locally.

SEHD has two ministers: the Minister for Health and Community Care and the Deputy Minister for Health and Community Care. The head of SEHD is also the chief executive of NHSScotland, and is accountable to ministers for the efficiency and performance of the service.

Scotland's chief medical officer is the Executive's principal medical adviser, with direct access to ministers. The CMO is also head of the Scottish Medical Civil Service. The post has direct involvement in developing health policy, including prevention, health promotion, health protection and harm reduction. The CMO has lead responsibility for issues such as clinical effectiveness, quality assurance, accreditation and research.

SEHD has directorates covering:
- nursing, midwifery and allied health professions
- primary care and community care
- healthcare policy and strategy
- finance
- health improvement
- workforce
- delivery

SEHD has 650 staff.

www.sehd.scot.nhs.uk

Special health boards
Seven special health boards provide services nationally.

Golden Jubilee National Hospital
Bought from the private sector in 2002, the hospital carries out only elective procedures in key specialties to reduce waiting times.
www.show.scot.nhs.uk/gjnh

NHS 24
Provides 24-hour telephone access (0845 242424) to medical advice from clinical professionals and acts as a referral point to local out-of-hours services.
www.nhs24.com

NHS Education for Scotland
Designs, commissions and provides training and lifelong learning for NHSScotland's workforce.
www.nes.scot.nhs.uk

Health Scotland
Supports organisations, policy-makers, communities and individuals to take action to improve health and reduce health inequalities. It combines many of the roles performed in England by the Healthcare Commission and NICE.
www.healthscotland.com

NHS Quality Improvement Scotland
The lead organisation in improving healthcare quality by setting, monitoring and reporting on standards and advising on clinical practice.
www.nhshealthquality.org

Scottish Ambulance Service
Employs over 3,000 staff.
www.scottishambulance.com

The State Hospitals Board for Scotland
Cares for mentally ill patients needing treatment under secure conditions.
www.tsh.scot.nhs.uk

National Services Scotland

NSS is the Common Services Agency for NHSScotland. A non-departmental public body, it provides:
- specialist legal services
- counter-fraud services
- health statistics
- screening programmes
- family health service payments, patient registration and monitoring of clinical standards.

It also oversees:
- Health Protection Scotland, which carries out surveillance of communicable diseases, environmental health hazards and public health
- Scottish Healthcare Supplies
- Scottish Health Service Centre, which provides conference facilities, event organising, library and information services
- Scottish National Blood Transfusion Service.

www.nhsnss.org

NHS boards

NHSScotland abolished trusts in 2004 in favour of local single-system working based on 14 (originally 15) NHS boards (11 mainland and three island boards). This was intended to instil shared aims, common values and clear lines of accountability while breaking down traditional barriers between primary and acute care. Trusts were initially replaced by 'operating divisions' within the boards, each with a divisional management team headed by a divisional chief executive. In most boards these divisions have since been absorbed into an integrated board structure, with community health partnerships replacing the primary care division and a chief officer to oversee operational issues. The SEHD stressed that boards had to delegate operational powers to divisions to avoid centralising control; boards concentrate on strategic leadership and performance management across the entire local NHS.

Without the sharp distinction between purchasers and providers that exists in the English NHS, the health service in Scotland has rejected any significant role for an internal market in healthcare. However, work is underway to establish a Scottish national tariff – a set of standard prices for hospital procedures to simplify service-level agreements between boards for certain national and regional specialist services. The tariff is intended to create an incentive for efficiency by encouraging benchmarking among boards, and improve the accuracy of financial data by ensuring better recording of cost and activity data. NHS boards may also contract with independent providers to increase capacity in certain areas of care.

NHS boards are mainly responsible for:
- protecting and improving their population's health
- delivering hospital, community and primary care services
- developing a local health plan to address health priorities and needs
- allocating resources according to the board's strategic objectives
- the performance management of the local health system.

Boards have a statutory duty to take part in regional and national planning as part of regional planning groups.

Each NHS board includes, as full non-executive directors:
- an employee director
- the chair of the area clinical forum
- the chair of the community health partnerships advisory forum
- a representative from the university medical school (where applicable)
- an elected council member from each local authority area covered by the board.

Community health partnerships

CHPs were set up in April 2005 to manage primary and community health services and replace the 79 local healthcare co-operatives. They number 36, with every NHS board having at least one, while the largest board – Greater Glasgow – has eight. CHPs act as a focus for integrating primary and specialist services locally, forging partnerships with local authorities and the voluntary sector. Several CHPs have developed particularly advanced partnership arrangements with local authority community care services, and have evolved into community health and care partnerships (CHCPs).

Boards are expected to devolve power and responsibility to frontline staff in CHPs. Each CHP has a director or general manager, as well as a chair who is usually a health board non-executive director. CHPs have evolved to replace the old primary care operating divisions within NHS boards, and are now the mechanism for designing, planning and delivering all community-based services. CHP directors and general managers are core members of a board's senior management team.

CHPs' current priorities are:
- improving access to primary care services
- taking a systematic approach to long-term conditions
- encouraging anticipatory care
- supporting people at home
- preventing avoidable hospital admissions
- providing more local diagnosis and treatment
- enabling discharge and rehabilitation
- improving specific health outcomes
- improving health and tackling inequalities.

In addition, the SEHD is encouraging CHPs to:
- act on patient/carer experiences
- agree and deliver joint outcomes
- integrate service delivery
- develop community infrastructure
- develop the workforce.

Managed clinical networks

Managed clinical networks for a wide range of conditions became well established in Scotland before the rest of the UK. They are defined as:

> linked groups of health professionals and organisations from primary, secondary and tertiary care, working in a co-ordinated manner, unconstrained by existing professional and health board boundaries, to ensure equitable provision of high-quality clinically effective services throughout Scotland.

They are seen as an important way of integrating systems of care and developing clinical leadership. Managed care networks are a development of the concept, designed to cross boundaries between the NHS and social work departments.

Key organisations

Scottish Health Council

The Scottish Health Council exists to ensure the views of patients and the public are properly taken into account by NHS boards. It assesses how boards are involving patients in decisions about health services, develops examples of best practice in public involvement and help patients to give feedback to boards about their experiences of services. Although part of NHS Quality Improvement Scotland (see page 165), the council has its own identity and responsibilities, with a national office in Glasgow and local offices in each board area, where most of its staff are based. Members of the community are being appointed to serve on a local advisory council for each NHS board area.
www.scottishhealthcouncil.org

Scottish Medicines Consortium (SMC)

The Scottish Medicines Consortium, an independent group within NHS Quality Improvement Scotland, advises NHSScotland on the clinical and cost-effectiveness of all newly licensed medicines, new formulations of existing medicines and all new conditions the medicines will treat. It has 34 members, including healthcare professionals from NHS boards, pharmaceutical industry representatives and lay members. The SMC has also compiled a database of 180 experts to advise on its decisions. The introduction of the SMC as a single advisory body has led to Scotland leading the UK in early, post-launch assessment of new medicines. It ensures that NHSScotland receives regular and standardised advice to enable it to introduce effective medicines as rapidly as possible. The SMC's decisions do not have statutory force, however, and it cannot insist that NHS boards prescribe a particular drug.
www.scottishmedicines.org

Strategy and policy

Bringing the NHS under the control of elected representatives in Scotland for the first time has resulted in new directions for the Scottish health service that in some respects are quite distinct from policies pursued by the NHS in England. For example, NHSScotland has explicitly rejected market-based reforms of the kind being introduced south of the border, and the Scottish Parliament voted in favour of providing free personal care for elderly people, for which charges are levied in England.

Key targets and priorities

In the policy paper *Fair to all, personal to each* the minister announced in 2004 'unprecedented measures' for NHSScotland to cut waiting times. This pledged that by the end of 2007:

- no patient would wait more than 18 weeks from GP referral to outpatient appointment
- no patient would wait more than 18 weeks from a decision to undertake treatment to the start of that treatment
- patients would be able to rely on shorter maximum waits for specific conditions:
  – 18 weeks from referral to completion of treatment for cataract surgery
  – four hours from arrival to discharge or transfer for accident and emergency treatment
  – 24 hours from admission to a specialist unit for hip surgery following fracture
  – 16 weeks from GP referral through a rapid-access chest pain clinic or equivalent, to cardiac intervention.

Vital statistics: life expectancy 2002/03 (years)

	Men	Women
England	76.2	80.7
Scotland	73.5	78.9
Wales	75.6	80.2
Northern Ireland	75.6	80.4

Source: UK health departments

Recent milestones in Scottish health policy

Designed to care
A 1997 white paper that announced primary care trusts and local healthcare co-ops were to be set up from 1999. PCTs were responsible for all primary and community health services, while local healthcare co-operatives (LHCCs) involved GPs in developing service provision.

Health Act 1999
This ended the purchaser–provider split in Scotland, cutting trusts from 46 to 28 and abolishing GP fundholding.

Our national health
The Scottish NHS plan, published in December 2000, establishing unified NHS boards from 2001, under which trusts became integrated into a single local system, though remaining separate legal entities.

Community Care and Health (Scotland) Act 2002
This Act enabled the NHS and local authorities to pool budgets for community care and created 'joint futures' management bodies for community care services. Provides legislative backing for implementing free nursing and personal care (see next page).

Partnership for care
A white paper, published in February 2003, that abolished trusts from 2004 and replaced LHCCs with community health partnerships.

Fair to all, personal to each – the next steps for NHSScotland
In December 2004, this set new targets for 'radical improvements' to the patient's journey through the system.

Delivering for health
Published in October 2005, this set new priorities for NHSScotland (see next page).

Spotlight on policy: free personal and nursing care

Uniquely in the UK, personal and nursing care services for people over 65 have been available free in Scotland since July 2002. Eligibility depends on a needs assessment by the local authority, but is irrespective of income, capital assets, marital status or any care contribution by an unpaid carer. Personal care is defined as including help with personal hygiene, continence management, eating, simple treatments and personal assistance tasks. The Executive is providing £169 million for the policy in 2007/08. A reference group, expected to report in 2007, is evaluating the policy and will examine the range of services provided, their quality, costs and the difference free personal care has made to people's lives. The policy appears to have strong public support in Scotland, with 75 per cent saying the state should pay for personal care for those who need it. It is estimated to have helped more than 50,000 people so far.

In 2006, the Scottish Parliament Health Committee's care inquiry report found teething problems in implementing the policy but overall judged it to have been a success.

In 2005, after the 14-month Kerr inquiry had produced detailed recommendations for shaping NHSScotland for the future, the SEHD published *Delivering for health*, an action plan based on the national framework for service change developed by the Kerr group. This seeks to secure the long-term sustainability of acute and specialist services, improve access to care and shift focus on to preventive and continuous care in local communities, with resources targeted on those with the greatest risk of ill-health. Key priorities over the next decade include:
- reducing health inequalities by providing deprived communities with enhanced primary care teams, resources to identify at-risk populations and early access to preventive interventions
- enabling people with long-term conditions to live healthier lives by increasing support for self-care, extending primary care, offering integrated and responsive specialist care and anticipating the needs of vulnerable people
- streaming planned care – separating dedicated A&E and planned care units to improve the predictability of workflow and resources, reducing cancellations. This will mean more local A&E units, backed by larger central units

- creating a national information and communication technology system including an electronic patient record to improve the integration, quality and productivity of NHSScotland.

The SEHD reported in 2006 that of its 62 targets, 49 had been achieved, 11 were on track, one had been delayed and one (recruiting an extra 600 consultants) looked unlikely to be achieved.

Further information
A partnership for a better Scotland – delivering our commitments, Scottish Executive, December 2006.

Financing NHSScotland

Sources of funding
General taxation and national insurance contributions form the main source of funding for NHSScotland, as they do for the NHS in the rest of the UK. Charges and receipts from land sales or other assets add comparatively small sums to the total. However, the Scottish Parliament is able to raise additional taxes, although it has yet to do so.

Resource allocation
UK Government spending reviews, which take place every two years and cover a three-year cycle, determine the amount of public expenditure available for Scotland. Increases to the Scottish budget are made according to the population-based 'Barnett formula', introduced in 1978 and modified slightly since devolution.

The Scottish Executive then decides how this sum should be allocated among its departments, subject to the Scottish Parliament's approval. The health and community care budget has three main elements:
- hospital and community health services and family health services expenditure – the largest item, which includes payments to GPs, dentists, pharmacists and optometrists; the GP drugs bill; the costs of primary, acute and community health services
- other health services – including the welfare foods scheme, research and public health
- community care – central government spending on grants to voluntary organisations and on the Scottish Commission for the Regulation of Care; most community care spending is incurred by local authorities.

Part of the budget is top-sliced to fund national projects and SEHD spending on national programmes such as nurse education and training. Then resources are allocated to NHS boards under two categories:
- cash-limited unified budget – spent on hospital and community health services, including GP prescribing, and forming the bulk of boards' discretionary allocation
- non-cash limited demand-led expenditure – spent on family health services provided by primary care contractors.

Allocations to boards are made using the Arbuthnott weighted capitation formula, devised in 2000. This is based on population characteristics, levels of deprivation and an adjustment for remoteness. Boards can carry forward underspending of up to 1 per cent of their budgets. The NHSScotland Resource Allocation Committee consulted on changes to the formula in 2006, and ministers are expected to make a final decision in 2007.

For 2006/07 NHS boards were given a general allocation of £6.4 billion, an average increase of 7.25 per cent. All boards received a standard increase of 6.75 per cent, with those below their Arbuthnott formula target allocation receiving more. NHS boards' spending was divided as follows:
- hospitals – 60 per cent
- family health services – 27 per cent
- community health services – 13 per cent.

In 2005/06, NHSScotland and the SEHD had a surplus of £70.6 million on their combined budget of £9 billion, all of it on capital funding – although two boards finished with deficits. NHSScotland and the SEHD had finished the previous year with a combined deficit of £32 million. Their combined budget for 2007/08 is £10 billion.

Further information
Overview of the financial performance of the NHS in Scotland 2005/06, Audit Scotland, December 2006.

Staffing and human resources

Staff numbers
A total of 153,996 people were employed in NHSScotland in September 2005 (the latest figures available) on a headcount basis. Since 1995 the workforce has grown by 16,849, an increase of 12 per cent.

In total there were:
- 14,133 doctors
- 2,695 dentists
- 65,816 nursing and midwifery staff
- 24,194 therapeutic, scientific, technical, pharmacy and ambulance staff
- 47,158 administrative and estates staff.

Staff in NHSScotland 2005

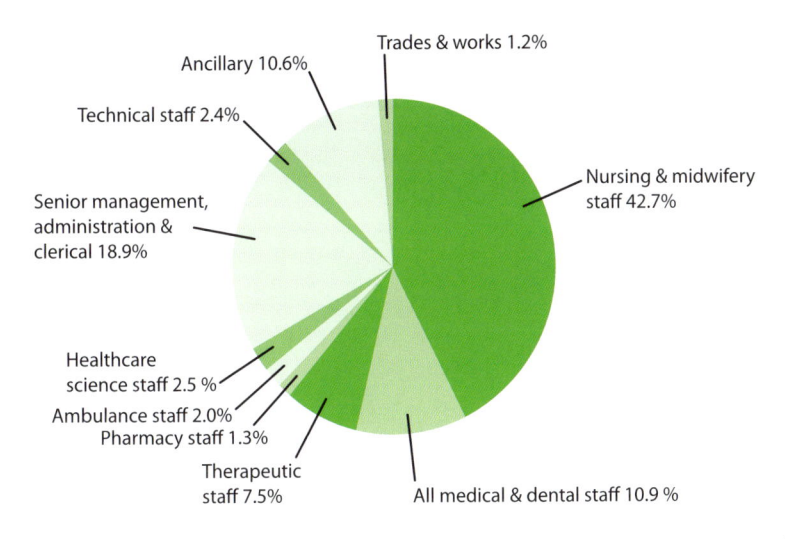

- Trades & works 1.2%
- Ancillary 10.6%
- Technical staff 2.4%
- Senior management, administration & clerical 18.9%
- Healthcare science staff 2.5%
- Ambulance staff 2.0%
- Pharmacy staff 1.3%
- Therapeutic staff 7.5%
- All medical & dental staff 10.9%
- Nursing & midwifery staff 42.7%

Source: NHS National Services Scotland

NHS staff: a cross-border comparison (2005)

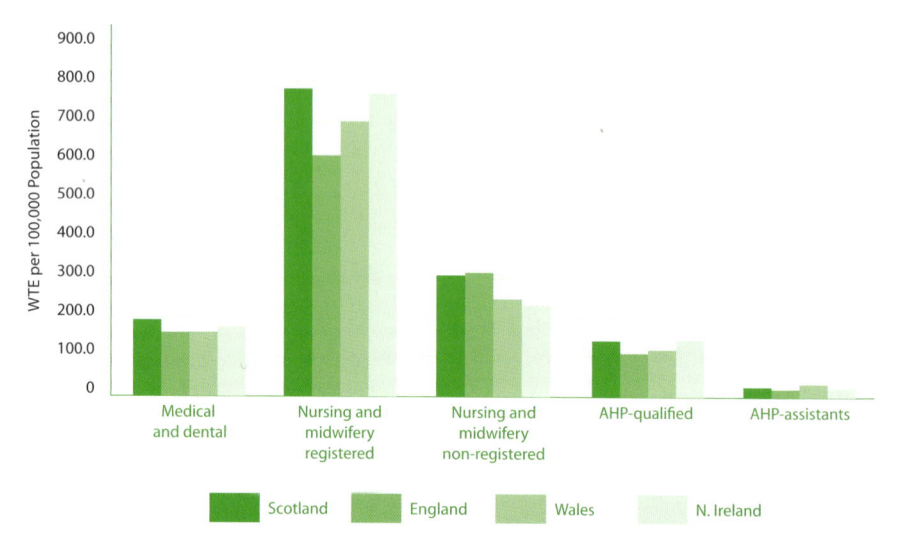

[Bar chart showing WTE per 100,000 Population across categories: Medical and dental, Nursing and midwifery registered, Nursing and midwifery non-registered, AHP-qualified, AHP-assistants, for Scotland, England, Wales, and N. Ireland]

Source: Scottish Executive Health Department

Workforce planning

NHSScotland published its first national workforce plan in 2006, detailing extra places for trainee GPs and hospital doctors and pledging to maintain numbers for pre-registration nursing and midwifery training. The rate of growth of NHSScotland's workforce is lower than the other UK countries', but its staff-to-population ratio is higher. Its workforce is also older than that of other UK countries.

Further information

National workforce plan 2006, Scottish Executive Health Department, December 2006.
Working for health: the workforce development action plan for NHSScotland, August 2002.

Staff Governance Standard

Our national health, the Scottish Executive's health plan published in 2000, committed the NHS to becoming Scotland's best employer. The core standards for human resources practice in NHSScotland are set out in the Staff Governance Standard, which all NHS organisations must adhere to. This entitles all staff to be:
- well informed
- appropriately trained

- involved in decisions that affect them
- treated fairly and consistently
- provided with an improved and safe working environment.

The standard is supplemented by a series of best practice guidelines published by the Partnership Information Network Board. Topics include dignity at work, equal opportunities, family-friendly policies, personal development and dealing with employee concerns. NHS employers are expected to implement these fully.

The NHSScotland staff opinion survey for 2006, in which a third of employees took part, found that 72 per cent felt their job made good use of their skills and abilities, 80 per cent were clear about what they were expected to achieve and 74 per cent felt positive about support from colleagues.

Local partnership forums

Each NHSScotland organisation has a local partnership forum to foster communication between staff, trade unions and managers. Each NHS board area has an area partnership forum. All NHS employers must develop a partnership agreement with staff and their representatives, which must contain – as a minimum – commitments to communication and consultation, access to information and board meetings and organisational change policies. Local partnership forums are mirrored nationally by the Scottish Partnership Forum, comprising senior NHS board managers, trade union national officers and health department representatives.

Every NHS board has an employee director as a full non-executive member. This is usually the elected staff representative from the local area partnership forum.

Information technology in NHSScotland

eHealth IM&T strategy

NHSScotland launched its National eHealth IM&T strategy in 2004. It is designed around the pledge in *Partnership for care* to 'deliver an integrated care record jointly managed by patients and professional NHS staff with in-built security of access governed by patient consent'.

It has four main components:
- local GP/specialty electronic patient records, such as a GP or A&E system, a diabetic or cancer record, linked if appropriate to the local integrated care record.
- local integrated care record: NHS board-wide information system holding test results, clinical letters and summaries of care contributions.
- national integrated care record: NHSScotland-wide based and holding copies of information from other national systems such as immunisation, as well as summaries of information from the local integrated care record.
- information shared between agencies – for example, under agreed protocols for care of the elderly or children.

Implementation is overseen by a National eHealth/IM&T Programme Board, chaired by the minister.

Audit Scotland found that NHSScotland did not know exactly how much it spent on IM&T overall, but noted that its estimated budget of £65 million revenue and £35 million capital in 2006/07 fell well short of the Wanless recommendation (see page 113) of 3 to 4 per cent of total health spend – which would have been £373 million. However, NHSScotland is planning substantial revenue growth in IM&T to over £100 million revenue and £40 million capital for 2007/08.

The NHS in England has its own national programme for IT, see page 133; NHS Wales also has its own approach, Informing Healthcare, see page 192.

Further information
Informed to care: managing IT to deliver information in the NHS in Scotland, Audit Scotland, November 2006.
National ehealth/IM&T strategy, NHSScotland, April 2004.

Scotland's Health on the Web (SHOW)
This website is the official gateway to online information about NHSScotland.
www.show.scot.nhs.uk

Care Services Improvement Partnership **CSIP**

10 High Impact Changes for Mental Health Services

In June 2006 the Care Services Improvement Partnership (CSIP) launched the 10 High Impact Changes for Mental Health Services.

The 10 High Impact Changes for Mental Health Services are:

1. Treat home based care and support as the norm for the delivery of mental health services
2. Improve flow of service users and carers across health and social care by improving access to screening and assessment
3. Manage variation in service user discharge processes
4. Manage variation in access to all mental health services
5. Avoid unnecessary contact for service users and provide necessary contact in the right care setting
6. Increase the reliability of interventions by designing care based on what is known to work and that service users and carers inform and influence
7. Apply a systematic approach to enable the recovery of people with long term conditions
8. Improve service user flow by removing queues
9. Optimise service user and carer flow through the service using an integrated care pathway approach, and
10. Redesign and extend roles in line with efficient service user and carer pathways to attract and retain an effective workforce.

Throughout 2007 we will continue to develop the evidence base that underpins the high impact changes. Our aim is to strengthen our understanding of service improvements that can demonstrate effective and efficient care delivery measured in terms of quality and value to service users, carers, providers and commissioners.

For more information about our work please telephone **01206 287544**, email *info@csip.org.uk* or visit *www.nimhe.csip.org.uk/10highimpactchanges*

High Impact Changes for Health and Social Care

CSIP are now also developing a set of changes that have the biggest positive impact in health and social care on achieving the 7 outcomes of adult social care (improved health and emotional well-being, improved quality of life, making a positive contribution, choice and control, freedom from discrimination, economic well-being and personal dignity).
We are currently collecting evidence throughout the country to determine what the changes are and will be launching them in January 2008.
The changes will provide a framework for service improvement and will support the implementation of the White Paper "Our health, our care, our say".

Visit *www.csip.org.uk/highimpactchanges forhealthandsocialcare*

We help to improve services and achieve better outcomes for children and families, adults and older people including those with mental health problems, physical or learning disabilities or people in the criminal justice system. We work with and are funded by **DH** Department of Health

10

The NHS in Wales

The structure of NHS Wales

National Assembly for Wales
The National Assembly for Wales opened in 1999 and has 60 elected members (AMs). The UK Parliament devolved to it power to pass secondary legislation. It can therefore develop and implement policies, make rules and regulations, set standards and issue guidance in areas that include health and social services, housing, local government, education and economic development. The Assembly can only do this within the basic framework of primary legislation that is made by the UK Parliament, but the Government of Wales Act 2006 will extend its powers further.

The Assembly provides democratic control of the management and performance of NHS Wales. It draws up strategic policies, sets priorities and allocates funds, but it is not able to raise extra taxes.

The Assembly's eight subject committees help develop policies and advise on budget allocations, as well as exercising scrutiny over ministers and legislation. Membership reflects the balance of political groups within the Assembly. The eight-member Health and Social Services Committee covers health and NHS Wales, social services and social care and food safety.

Among the Assembly's seven standing committees, the Audit Committee scrutinises the expenditure of NHS Wales by examining reports on its accounts prepared by the Auditor General for Wales. The Wales Audit Office, created in 2005, combines the offices of the Audit Commission and the National Audit Office in Wales.

Regional committees represent the needs and interests of their localities, and convey issues of local concern to the full Assembly and to the subject committees. There are five, made up of members from the relevant constituency and electoral region.

The Wales Office, led by the Secretary of State for Wales, represents Welsh interests in the UK Government and Parliament.

Further information
National Assembly for Wales www.wales.gov.uk/index.htm
Wales Office www.walesoffice.gov.uk
Wales Audit Office www.wao.gov.uk

Welsh Assembly Government
The Welsh Assembly Government is the Assembly's executive body, led by the First Minister and an eight-strong cabinet that includes a Minister for Health and Social Services. The First Minister is elected by AMs, and is therefore usually the leader of the largest party. Assembly elections are held every four years, the last being in May 2007. Of the Assembly's 60 members, 40 are elected in constituencies using the first-past-the-post system; the other 20 are elected to represent the five regions of Wales.

Health and Social Care Department
The Health and Social Care Department was established in 2004 with responsibility for:
- advising the Assembly on health and social care policies and strategies
- contributing to health and social care legislation
- funding the NHS and other health and social care bodies
- managing and supporting the delivery of health and social care services
- monitoring and promoting improvements in service delivery.

Other responsibilities include research and development, finance, human resources, information management and technology, capital and estates. The department's head is also chief executive of NHS Wales and the accounting officer for the health service. The department's constituent parts are:
- community, primary care and health service directorate
- quality, standards and safety improvement directorate
- resource directorate
- children's health and social care directorate
- older people and long-term care policy directorate
- performance and operations directorate
- strategy unit
- organisational development and training team
- NHS human resources.

Regional offices
Three regional offices – for North Wales, Mid and West Wales, and South and East Wales – act as agents for the chief executive of NHS Wales on a day-to-day basis. They hold to account the chief executives of the 36 statutory NHS bodies, and manage their performance through the performance improvement framework and accountability agreements. The chief executive of NHS Wales and the regional directors also conduct an annual review process.

Local health boards (LHBs)
Local health boards' main roles are:
- corporate and clinical governance
- commissioning and providing primary and community care health services
- commissioning secondary care services
- improving the health of communities
- partnership
- public engagement.

There are 22 LHBs, all of which are coterminous with unitary local authorities. Each LHB has its own board and management team. LHBs receive 75 per cent of the NHS Wales budget. LHBs are expected to take the lead in ensuring partnership and joined-up working with local authorities – including services such as housing and education – and the independent and voluntary sectors. Each LHB and local unitary authority in conjunction with other partners is expected to produce a strategy for the health and well-being of the public.

NHS trusts

There are 14 NHS trusts in Wales, including the all-Wales ambulance trust. They are key providers of services, managing 135 hospitals and 15,000 beds. Wales has one main teaching hospital, the University Hospital of Wales based in Cardiff, as well as a network of district general and community hospitals. Half a million people – a sixth of the population – will have a hospital stay in any given year. Most trust income derives from providing services commissioned by LHBs under long-term agreements. Trusts are held accountable for their performance under these agreements.

Community health councils

CHCs are statutory lay organisations with rights to information about, access to, and consultation with all NHS organisations on behalf of the public. There are 20 CHCs in Wales. In 2004 the Welsh Assembly Government strengthened CHCs' powers and responsibilities to give the public a stronger voice and better advice on NHS issues. Changes included:
- an independent complaints advocacy service across Wales
- rights to visit GP and dental surgeries, opticians and pharmacies
- rights to visit private nursing homes where NHS patients are being treated.

A statutory body, the Board of Community Health Councils in Wales, represents CHCs, gathers information of concern to patients and reports it to the Assembly's Health and Social Services Committee. It also liaises with the Department of Health in London on cross-border concerns and funding problems beyond the Assembly's scope.

Further information
Board of Community Health Councils in Wales: **www.patienthelp.wales.nhs.uk**

Health Commission Wales (Specialist Services)

This executive agency is a specialist health services commissioning body responsible for:
- tertiary and other highly specialised services throughout Wales
- advising NHS Wales on commissioning specialised secondary and regional services
- providing dedicated guidance, support and facilitation for acute services commissioning
- being the first source of arm's-length independent advice and guidance on difficult issues relating to specialist services.

www.wales.gov.uk/healthcommission

NHS Wales Business Services Centre (BSC)

BSC, part of Powys LHB, provides shared-services support to LHBs and independent contractors such as GPs, pharmacists, dentists and opticians. It has four departments:

- finance – processing invoices, producing financial accounts, providing ledger management, as well as counter-fraud and management information
- contractor services – administrative support for primary care contracts, patient and clinical services, business support, payment processing and post payment verification
- information management and technology – providing a corporate information service, ICT infrastructure design and support, primary care ICT support and information governance
- human resources – developing HR policies, recruitment and selection, training and development, organisational development and HR advice and support to staff.

www.bsc.wales.nhs.uk

Healthcare Inspectorate Wales

HIW, launched in 2004, works closely with the Healthcare Commission (see page 82). It monitors, reviews and investigates standards in Welsh NHS bodies. This includes:

- inspecting NHS bodies and service providers against national standards, agreements and clinical governance guidance in Wales
- assessing management arrangements for clinical governance and NHS services
- assessing the quality of NHS services across agencies and sectors using, for example, networks and patient journey tracking.

HIW has rights to enter and inspect premises, as well as powers to require documents and information.

www.hiw.wales.gov.uk

Welsh Innovations in Healthcare (WIsH)

WIsH's purpose is to provide the NHS in Wales with advice and support in maximising the potential of ideas, innovations and intellectual property generated by NHS organisations and their staff. These fall into two main categories:
- service innovations – usually new or improved ways of delivering services, such as new care pathways
- technology innovations – new or improved ideas for medical devices, therapeutics and software.

WIsH has prepared intellectual property policies for trusts and provided training for NHS research and development managers. It has also identified several healthcare innovations that have significant commercial potential.

www.wishnhswales.org.uk

Organisations spanning England and Wales

Organisations whose remit covers both England and Wales include:
- Healthcare Commission (see page 82)
- National Institute for Health and Clinical Excellence (see page 87)
- National Patient Safety Agency (see page 88)
- Health Protection Agency (see page 156)
- NHS Direct (see page 43)
- Medicines and Healthcare Products Regulatory Agency (see page 215).

Key organisations: public health in Wales

Office of the Chief Medical Officer
The Office of the Chief Medical Officer (OCMO) leads on policy and programmes for protecting and improving health and reducing inequalities. It also provides professional and medical advice to ministers, the Health and Social Care Department and other parts of the Welsh Assembly Government. OCMO consists of:
- public health strategy division – which takes an overarching approach to improving health and reducing health inequalities
- health promotion division – responsible for developing and delivering evidence-based health promotion policy, strategy and programmes
- public health protection division – whose responsibilities include policy on communicable disease control, vaccination and immunisation and environmental health
- health professionals group – small specialist divisions and senior medical officers provide professional and medical advice to the First Minister, Minister for Health and Social Services and other areas of the Welsh Assembly Government.

National Public Health Service (NPHS) and the Wales Centre for Health (WCH)
NPHS draws together most of the public health functions previously provided by Wales's five health authorities until they were replaced by LHBs in 2003. It offers public health advice and expertise mainly to LHBs, and is structured around the three regional offices, each of which has a regional public health director.

WCH is closely linked to the work on public health. Its main functions are to:
- collate public health data and evidence and advise policy-makers
- co-ordinate surveillance of health trends and carry out risk assessments
- open up wider public health training in Wales and build a multidisciplinary workforce of specialists and practitioners.

Further information
Office of the Chief Medical Officer: www.cmo.wales.gov.uk
National Public Health Service: www.nphs.wales.nhs.uk
Wales Centre for Health: www.wch.wales.nhs.uk

Strategy and policy

Although the NHS in Wales has had slightly different policy and structural arrangements from England for most of its existence, these have diverged more markedly since devolution in an attempt to find distinctively Welsh solutions for specifically Welsh problems. Wales has some of the UK's highest rates of cancer, heart disease and deprivation, while part of its population suffers the worst health status in Europe.

Key targets and priorities

In 2005 the *Designed for life* white paper set out a ten-year vision for NHS Wales that would transform it 'from the national illness service it currently is into a truly national health service', and involve significant change 'probably in every hospital, GP practice and every social services department'. Three strategic frameworks, each covering three years, would achieve this. Each set targets in key policy areas:

- 2005–08: redesigning care
- 2008–11: delivering higher standards
- 2011–14: ensuring full engagement.

Vital statistics: hospital beds 2002/03 (per 1,000 population)

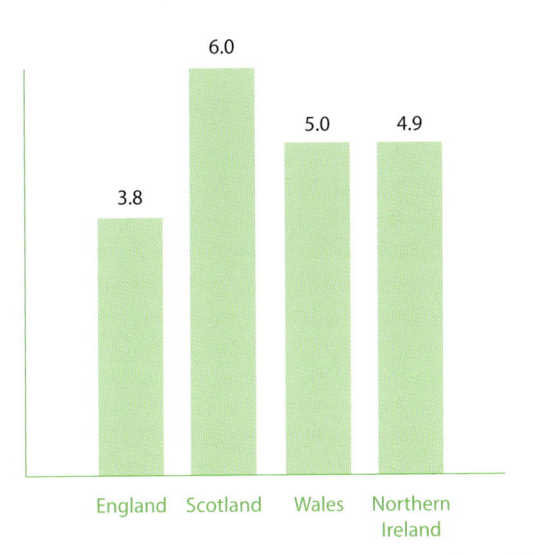

England	Scotland	Wales	Northern Ireland
3.8	6.0	5.0	4.9

Source: UK health departments

Recent milestones in Welsh health policy

Putting patients first
Published in 1998, this abolished GP fundholding in Wales and set up local health groups as part of the existing five health authorities.

Better health, better Wales
Also published in 1998, this explicitly linked poverty and ill-health.

Improving health in Wales – a plan for the NHS with its partners
The Welsh NHS plan published in January 2001, this proposed new structures: establishing the Health and Social Care Department, three regional offices and several other all-Wales bodies, as well as replacing the five health authorities and local health groups with 22 local health boards.

Review of health and social care in Wales: the Wanless Report
The Welsh Assembly Government appointed Derek Wanless to examine how resources could be translated into reform and improved performance in health and social care. In July 2003 he recommended:
- a radical redesign for health and social care services
- an evidence-based approach to best practice and improving system performance
- developing capacity outside acute hospitals
- more public and patient involvement
- stronger performance-management systems.

Designed for life: creating world-class health and social care for Wales in the 21st century
Updating *Improving health in Wales*, this is the Welsh Assembly Government's vision for the NHS up to 2015, influenced by the Wanless Report and published in May 2005.

Targets to be achieved by 2008 include:
- a wait of no more than 26 weeks from GP or dental referral to treatment (including diagnostic and therapy treatment)
- 95 per cent of all patients to spend less than four hours in A&E until admission, transfer or discharge
- all NHS trusts to have an approved health promotion strategy covering services and staff
- access to services for HIV and sexually transmitted infection and routine contraception advice within two working days.

In addition:
- 'significant capital investment' will help remodel mental health services
- chronic disease-management services will be remodelled to develop a new care programme approach
- children's and young people's services will be improved with better partnership working
- older people's services will be integrated
- cancer services will be reconfigured.

Further information
Designed for life: creating world-class health and social care for Wales in the 21st century, NHS Wales, May 2005.

Spotlight on policy: free prescriptions

The Welsh Assembly Government abolished all prescription charges in April 2007, having reduced them progressively since 2001. Wales is the only part of the UK to adopt this policy; in England charges are currently £6.85. Only those with a GP and a pharmacist in Wales can take advantage of the scheme. It is estimated the policy will benefit about 1.5 million people who are not exempt from charges, and cost about £30 million a year.

Financing NHS Wales

Sources of funding
General taxation and national insurance contributions form the main source of funding for NHS Wales, as they do for the NHS in the rest of the UK. Charges and receipts from land sales or other assets add comparatively small sums to the total. The Welsh Assembly, unlike the Scottish Parliament, is unable to raise additional taxes.

Resource allocation
UK Government spending reviews, which take place every two years and cover a three-year cycle, determine the amount of public expenditure available for Wales. Increases to the Welsh block grant are made according to the population-based 'Barnett formula', introduced in 1978 and modified slightly since devolution.

The Welsh Assembly Government then decides how this sum should be allocated among its departments, subject to the Assembly's approval. The health budget comprises seven expenditure groups:
- LHBs and NHS trusts – funds allocated to LHBs for purchasing care from trusts
- education and training – mainly for doctors and nurses
- family health services – GP pay and prescribing costs, plus dental and ophthalmic costs
- health improvement – public health initiatives, including immunisation
- health promotion – in schools, workplaces, local communities and the NHS
- food standards – funding the Welsh Executive of the Food Standards Agency
- welfare foods – free milk to children and expectant mothers on income support.

Allocations to LHBs are made using the 'Townsend formula' devised in 2001. Its principal aim is to curb growth in health inequalities by better targeting NHS resources into areas of greatest need.

Health communities – LHBs, trusts, GPs and others – draw up service and financial frameworks (SaFFs) every year to match their planned activity to available resources. SaFFs are published in March, and are expected to achieve the Welsh Assembly Government's national priorities as well as local ones. They assist joint planning and provide a basis for performance management throughout the year. LHBs also make long-term service agreements with NHS trusts for the work they wish to commission from them – the main method by which trusts receive the funding that makes up their budgets.

In 2007/08, health and social services account for £5.5 billion of the Welsh Assembly Government's £14.6 billion budget, an increase of about 7 per cent on the previous year. It began 2006/07 with a deficit of £30 million from 2005/06 and previously outstanding debt of £83 million that must be repaid by 2009.

Further information
Is the NHS in Wales managing within its available resources? Wales Audit Office, April 2006.

Staffing and human resources

Staff numbers
A total of 94,300 people worked in NHS Wales in 2005 (the latest figures available) on a whole-time equivalent basis. Of these, over 68,000 people were directly employed by NHS Wales, a 3 per cent increase on 2004. More than three-quarters were women.

In total there were:
- 4,684 hospital doctors and dentists
- 28,152 nurses, midwives and health visitors
- 9,699 scientific, therapeutic and technical staff
- 8,584 healthcare assistants and other support staff
- 15,421 administration and estates staff
- 1,394 ambulance staff.

In addition, there were 1,816 GPs, 1,024 general dental practitioners and 4,171 practice support staff.

Workforce planning
Designed for life noted that NHS Wales needed a new process for workforce planning and commissioning education – a strengthened, integrated and more streamlined model of whole-system workforce redesign. *Designed to work* aims to help bring about the staffing changes needed to achieve the goals of *Designed for life*, particularly cultural change and engaging clinical leaders. It contains a three-year action plan to be reviewed and modified at the end of 2008.

Further information
Designed to work: a workforce strategy to deliver Designed for life, Welsh Assembly Government, July 2006.
Making the connections: connecting the workforce: the workforce challenge for health, Welsh Assembly Government, July 2005.

Key organisation: National Leadership and Innovation Agency for Healthcare

NLIAH was set up in 2005 to help build leadership capacity and capability underpinned by technology, innovation, leading-edge thinking and best practice. Its programme includes work on:
- innovative models of clinical leadership
- modernisation assessments across health communities
- collecting and disseminating best practice and ensuring its uptake.

Its 2006/07 programme focused on chronic disease management. NLIAH's workforce development, education and contracting unit covers workforce planning, NHS careers information, standards setting, continued professional development and lifelong learning. Monthly NLIAH e-bulletins provide information on the progress.
www.nliah.wales.nhs.uk

Information technology in NHS Wales

NHS Wales's IT strategy, Informing Healthcare, was launched in 2003. It will achieve its aims through a series of planned and agreed service improvement projects.

Informing Healthcare focuses on:

Single patient record
Every patient will have a single electronic health record, with the eventual aim of fully integrated health and social care records.

Workforce empowerment
All NHS Wales staff will be given access to new skills allowing them to use the new systems. Training will range from basic IT and information management skills to more specialist health informatics skills. This will enable them to take advantage of new productivity tools and computerised business support services. Employees will have access through the new HR system to their own staff record.

Patient empowerment
By providing better information about treatments, risks and benefits, patients will be able to play a more active role in decision-making about their treatments, and their satisfaction with services should increase.

Service improvement
Modernisation and IT in healthcare have not been well integrated. The Informing Healthcare strategy argues that they must be closely aligned both strategically and in practice.

Knowledge management
Knowledge management is concerned with collecting, making best use of and providing access to necessary information while minimising the collection of information that brings little benefit.

Informing Healthcare is expected to invest £91 million over its first three years of operation, 2004–07. A national programme team has been set up, in addition to local teams in trusts and primary care.

Further information
Informing Healthcare: www.wales.nhs.uk/ihc

Health of Wales Information Service (HOWIS)
This website is the official gateway to online information about NHS Wales.
www.wales.nhs.uk

The NHS in England has its own national programme for IT, see page 133; NHSScotland also has its own approach, eHealth IM&T strategy, see page 177.

11

The NHS in Northern Ireland

The structure of the NHS in Northern Ireland

Since 1972 the NHS in Northern Ireland has been integrated with social services and is known as the Health and Personal Social Services (HPSS).

Northern Ireland Assembly

The Northern Ireland Assembly was established as a result of the Good Friday Agreement of 1998. It was elected later that year, operated in shadow form without government powers until full devolution in December 1999, but was then suspended in October 2002. Recalled in May 2006, under the St Andrew's Agreement it sat as a 'transitional Assembly' whose sole purpose was to prepare for the restoration of full devolution after elections in March 2007.

When the Assembly sat from 1999 until 2002, it had full legislative and executive authority for 'transferred matters', which included areas such as health, social services, education and agriculture. In addition, it may at a later date take responsibility for 'reserved matters', such as policing and criminal law. 'Excepted matters' remain the UK Parliament's responsibility, and include defence, foreign policy and taxation.

The Assembly has 108 members (MLAs), six from each of Northern Ireland's 18 Westminster constituencies. A First Minister and a Deputy First Minister are elected to lead the ten-strong Executive Committee of Ministers. They have to stand for election jointly, and to be elected must have cross-community support. The parties elected to the Assembly choose ministerial portfolios and select ministers in proportion to their party strength. The Executive Committee brings forward proposals for new legislation in the form of Executive Bills for the Assembly to consider. It also sets out a programme for government each year, with an agreed budget for approval by the Assembly.

Ten cross-party statutory committees have power to examine, debate and recommend changes to the Northern Ireland departments' policies and decisions. This includes, for example, how money is shared and spent. The Health, Social Services and Public Safety Committee advises and assists the Minister of Health, Social Services and Public Safety to formulate policy and undertakes scrutiny, policy development and consultation. It has 11 members.

Among the Assembly' six standing committees, the 11-strong Public Accounts Committee's remit is to consider accounts covering the NHS in Northern Ireland. The committee has the power 'to send for persons, papers and records'.

The Secretary of State for Northern Ireland, who is a Westminster MP and member of the UK Government, assumes responsibilities for the Northern Ireland departments if the Assembly is suspended.
www.niassembly.gov.uk

Northern Ireland Executive

The Executive forms the government of Northern Ireland and comprises ten departments plus the Office of the First Minister and Deputy First Minister. Each department is headed by a minister who sits on the Assembly's Executive Committee. While devolution was suspended, the departments were run by the UK Government's Northern Ireland Office (NIO), headed by the Secretary of State for Northern Ireland and four other ministers.

Further information
Northern Ireland Executive: www.northernireland.gov.uk
Northern Ireland Office: www.nio.gov.uk

Department of Health, Social Services and Public Safety (DHSSPS)

While devolution was suspended, the Assembly's Minister of Health, Social Services and Public Safety was replaced by a parliamentary under-secretary of state at the NIO. This minister is also responsible for security, policing and prisons.

The DHSSPS is responsible for:
- health and personal social services – including policy and legislation for hospitals, family practitioner services, community health and personal social services
- public health – policy and legislation to promote and protect the health and well-being of Northern Ireland's population
- public safety – policy and legislation for the Fire Authority, food safety and emergency planning.

The department's permanent secretary presides over:
- Primary, Secondary and Community Care Group
- Planning and Resources Group – which negotiates and manages financial resources, departmental staffing and information systems support for the DHSSPS and HPSS bodies. It is also responsible for the HPSS's strategic plan, ambulance services, fire services and emergency planning
- Strategic Planning and Modernisation Group – responsible for the HPSS reform and service improvement programmes; it also manages the HPSS capital investment programme and regional strategy for health and social well-being
- five professional groups – for medical and allied services, Social Services Inspectorate, Nursing and Midwifery Advisory Group, dental services and pharmaceutical advices and services.
- Health Estates – an executive agency that determines policy on estate issues, as well as providing expert advice and consultancy services.

The DHSSPS employs 1,016 people and is by far the largest Northern Ireland department, accounting for two-fifths of the Northern Ireland budget.

www.dhsspsni.gov.uk

A system in transition: restructuring Northern Ireland health and social services

At present in the HPSS, there are:
- four health and social services boards, which assess needs and commission services
- 19 health and social services trusts, which provide health and social services as commissioned by the four boards and their local health and social care groups
- 15 local health and social care groups, set up as committees of the boards in 2002 to replace GP fundholding
- five regional service bodies including the Central Services Agency, the Health Promotion Agency and the Blood Transfusion Agency
- four health and social service councils, which represent users' views and provide independent oversight.

At the end of 2005, following a province-wide review of public administration, the Northern Ireland Health Minister announced major reforms of health and social services, reducing the number of organisations from 47 to 18. The plans include:
- a much smaller DHSSPS with about 500 staff will set strategic policy and longer-term targets, and manage the performance of the strategic authority
- a Health and Social Services Authority (HSSA) to replace the four health and social services boards, commission services on a region-wide basis and performance-manage the new trusts by April 2008
- the 18 health and social services trusts reduced to five, with the ambulance service remaining a separate trust; the new trusts to promote links between hospitals and community-based services, as well as integration across professions, geographical areas and between health and social services
- seven local commissioning groups – driven by GPs and primary care professionals – will act as local offices of the HSSA, which will be established by April 2008, taking on some of the roles from the four boards and their 15 local health and social care groups, which will be abolished; the local commissioning groups will be coterminous with the proposed seven new district councils, and commission services from trusts
- one Patient and Client Council replacing the existing four health and social services councils.

A reconfiguration programme board headed by the permanent secretary is leading implementation of the reforms. A public service commission has been set up by the Government to advise on safeguarding staff interests and smoothing the transition to the new organisations arising out of the review of public administration.

The five new integrated trusts have existed in shadow form since September 2006, and were formally established in April 2007. Consultation on the legislative changes needed to set up the HSSA opened in early 2007.

HPSS: new structure

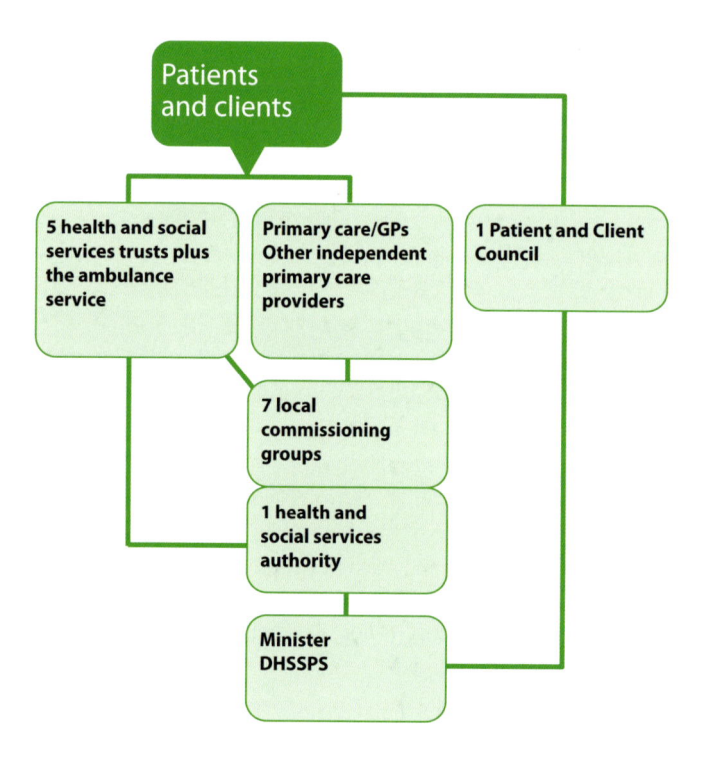

- Patients and clients
  - 5 health and social services trusts plus the ambulance service
  - Primary care/GPs Other independent primary care providers
    - 7 local commissioning groups
    - 1 health and social services authority
      - Minister DHSSPS
  - 1 Patient and Client Council

Source: Northern Ireland Department of Health, Social Services and Public Safety

Strategy and policy

Given Northern Ireland's unique geographical and political circumstances within the UK, it is to be expected that the NHS there has distinct characteristics – most notably that health and social care are integrated. While spending per head on health and social care is higher in Northern Ireland than in England, outputs and outcomes lag behind. Although this may be partly due to inefficiency, and therefore perhaps susceptible to reform, other reasons may include better quality of provision, the need to maintain hospitals in rural locations and the higher costs of delivering services in deprived areas.

Key targets and priorities

The DHSSPS develops an annual priorities-for-action document based on its public service agreement (PSA). Boards respond with health and well-being investment plans, which set out how they will meet the PSA goals. Then each trust produces a trust delivery plan which sets out how it will use its resources.

The DHSSPS's Draft Priorities and Budget 2006–08 included these PSA targets:
- reduce the maximum waiting time for patients needing inpatient, day case or outpatient treatment to six months by March 2010
- reduce the death rate from circulatory diseases by at least 20 per cent in people under 75 by 2010
- increase five-year survival rates for the main cancers including breast, colorectal and lung (excluding non-melanoma skin cancers) by 5 per cent by 2010.
- reduce the standardised suicide rate by 10 per cent by 2008
- reduce the proportion of adult smokers to 22 per cent or less, with a reduction in prevalence among manual groups to 27 per cent or less, by 2011
- by 2010 improve the quality of life and independence of people in need so that 45 per cent of all who require community services are supported, as necessary, in their homes (40 per cent by 2007)
- by 2008 all patients who request a clinical appointment through their general practice for other than emergencies to be able to see an appropriate primary care professional within two working days.

Recent milestones in Northern Ireland health policy

Investing for health
Published in 2002, this noted that health and well-being is largely determined by the social, economic, physical and cultural environment. The Executive identified health improvement as one of five overarching priorities in its programme for government. This DHSSPS strategy document sought to shift emphasis from treating ill-health to preventing it. It contained a framework for action to improve health and well-being and reduce health inequalities based on partnership among departments, public bodies, local communities, voluntary bodies, district councils and social partners.

Developing better services: modernising hospitals and reforming structures
Under the programme that resulted from this consultation document published in June 2002, Northern Ireland's 15 acute hospitals were replaced by a network of nine acute hospitals supported by seven local hospitals, with additional local hospitals in other locations as appropriate. The role of hospitals is to support community-based care services in promoting health and well-being.

A healthier future: a twenty-year vision for health and well-being in Northern Ireland 2005–2025
Published in December 2004, this identifies key policy directions, actions and outcomes that will contribute to achieving the vision. It is built around five cross-cutting themes: investing for health and well-being; involving people; teams which deliver; responsive and integrated services and improving quality. A key element is reforming HPSS planning to become more integrated. Actions identified are intended to support implementation of *Investing for health*. Tackling chronic diseases and socio-economic disadvantage is the strategy's main focus.

Recent milestones in Northern Ireland health policy continued

Independent review of health and social care services in Northern Ireland: the Appleby Report

In the manner of the Wanless Reports in England and Wales this report, published in August 2005, set out to examine the likely future resource needs of Northern Ireland's health and social services. It concluded that 'a significant increase in resources is required in the coming years, but with slower growth thereafter', but also that 'a significant underlying reason for current problems with the Northern Ireland health and social care sector relates to the use of resources rather than the amount of resources available'.

Vital statistics: inpatient admissions 2002/03 (per 1,000 population)

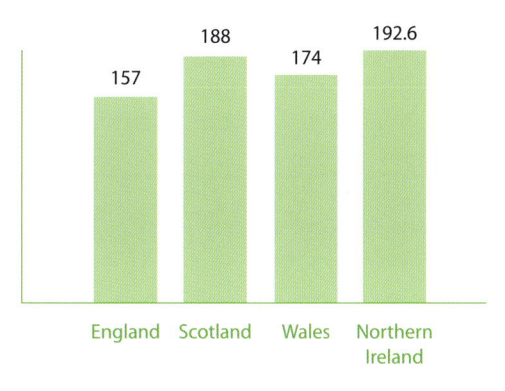

England	Scotland	Wales	Northern Ireland
157	188	174	192.6

Source: UK health departments

Financing the HPSS in Northern Ireland

Sources of funding

General taxation and national insurance contributions form the main source of funding for the HPSS in Northern Ireland, as they do for the NHS in the rest of the UK. Charges and receipts from land sales or other assets add comparatively small sums to the total. The Northern Ireland Assembly, unlike the Scottish Parliament, is unable to raise additional taxes.

Resource allocation

Under devolution, the Northern Ireland Executive sets targets for each of its departments in its annual programme for government.

Once the Chancellor has announced the Northern Ireland settlement, each department submits a position report with its financial requirements to the Department of Finance and Personnel (DFP) and Office of the First Minister. The DFP drafts a budget, which the Assembly considers alongside the draft programme for government. The Executive then revises the budget before deciding final allocations, which the Assembly debates and votes on.

The Minister for Health, Social Services and Public Safety then decides in detail how to allocate the department's resources for the coming year. The bulk is allocated to the boards to commission services from the trusts.

Allocations are made according to a weighted capitation formula which includes factors for demography, social deprivation and rurality. The allocation covers social services as well as health. The formula has been developed incrementally since the mid-1990s by the capitation formula review group. Some distinctive additional needs indicators are used in Northern Ireland, notably receipt of family credit and for maternity services, no previous births and multiple births.

The DHSSPS budget is divided among:
- hospital and community health services
- personal social services
- family health services.

The DHSSPS has the largest budget of any Northern Ireland department: in 2006/07 it was £3.5 billion. Of this, £2.3 billion was spent on hospital care, community health and personal social services, and £706 million on family practitioner services.

Further information
Strategic resources framework 2006/07, DHSSPS, December 2006.

Staffing and human resources

Staff numbers
In March 2005 the HPSS employed 57,293 people either full-time or part-time. This accounted for 9.5% of all in employment in Northern Ireland. These included:
- 3,413 medical and dental staff
- 15,638 qualified nurses and midwives
- 6,386 professional and technical staff
- 5,022 social services staff
- 889 ambulance staff
- 13,017 administrative and clerical staff
- 7,712 ancillary and general staff.

In addition, about 1,000 GPs work in Northern Ireland. In terms of headcount, staff increased by 23.6 per cent between 1996 and 2005.

Workforce planning
The DHSSPS's human resource directorate provides advice and guidance to HPSS employers on pay and terms and conditions of employment for health and social care staff. The directorate comprises:
- education and training unit
- HPSS superannuation branch
- pay and employment unit
- workforce planning unit.

In 2004 the Department of Finance and Personnel produced a pay and workforce strategy for the Northern Ireland Executive departments with a major focus on health. But unlike other aspects of health and social care, where distinct Northern Ireland policies are developed, on staff pay and conditions Northern Ireland tends to mirror the position in the rest of the UK.

2

Part 2: Gazetteer

The NHS: a brief history

Before the NHS
At the beginning of the 20th century, a network of charitable, voluntary and local authority hospitals had developed, but it was inadequate for the needs of a rapidly growing population. The charitable and voluntary hospitals dealt mainly with serious illnesses, while municipal health services comprised maternity hospitals, hospitals for infectious diseases like smallpox and tuberculosis and hospitals for elderly, mentally ill and mentally handicapped people.

The social reformer, Beatrice Webb, is often credited with being the first to call for a national health service, in 1909. A compromise was achieved in the 1911 National Insurance Act, under which wage-earners below a certain income received sickness benefit and treatment from doctors who contracted their services to local 'panels'. Workers' families were not covered. Outside the scheme, medical treatment had to be paid for – often according to what the patient could afford. As a result, many hospitals were brought to the brink of financial ruin.

Over the next 30 years, several developments paved the way for the NHS. In 1919 the Ministry of Health was established, and a Scottish Board of Health created to improve public health and encourage research, treatment and medical training. In the following year, the Dawson Report called for a single authority to oversee a comprehensive medical treatment system. Gradually throughout the 1920s and

1930s, the idea of a national system of publicly funded healthcare began to gain momentum.

With the outbreak of war it became a national priority, and the Emergency Medical Service was set up, giving the Government control over voluntary and municipal hospitals as well as responsibility for their funding. In 1942 the Beveridge Report described a vision for welfare reform based on eradication of the five giants of idleness, squalor, hunger, disease and ignorance. The coalition Government's 1944 white paper stated that the aims of a new health service would be:

> to ensure that in future every man and woman and child can rely on getting all the advice and treatment and care which they may need in matters of personal health; that what they get shall be the best medical and other facilities available; that their getting these shall not depend on whether they can pay for them, or any other factor irrelevant to the real need.

Early days

After the war, the Attlee Government's blueprint for the NHS described a public service more ambitious than any other western democracy's. It was to be universal – covering everyone; comprehensive – offering 'all necessary forms of healthcare'; and free at the point of use – funded from taxes. The proposal aroused widespread public enthusiasm, and for many enabled access to specialist services from which they had been excluded. The then Health Minister, Aneurin Bevan, called it 'the most civilised achievement of modern government'. The country was convinced it was creating 'the finest health service in the world'.

The NHS began throughout the UK on 5 July 1948. All voluntary and municipal hospitals were nationalised and overseen in England by 14 regional hospital boards, supported by 35 teaching hospital boards, which reported directly to the Ministry of Health. These boards supervised 400 hospital management committees, while 117 executive councils ran primary care services; local authorities were responsible for community care. Hospital doctors, nurses and other staff became state employees, although GPs remained independent and contracted their services to the NHS.

In theory, Bevan's system was intended to allow provision to meet demand. But initial funding failed to take account of the problems the service inherited, the unfair distribution of resources or the need to raise standards. No one had anticipated how demand would explode once long unmet needs could be satisfied. Soon the Government introduced dental, optical and prescription charges.

With funding capped during its formative years, the NHS had to rely on efficiency gains and increases in charges to expand services. The Conservative Government commissioned an inquiry into NHS costs, but the 1956 Guillebaud Report found little justification for charges and called for more resources to modernise hospitals and community care – to no avail. The NHS's rate of growth fell behind other health services, yet by 1958 *The Times* could declare: 'The nation has good reason to be proud of the NHS.'

Reorganisation and reform

In 1962, Health Minister Enoch Powell's Hospital Plan proposed developing district general hospitals in England to serve populations of 125,000 in recognition that the NHS's ageing and neglected infrastructure was inadequate for modern healthcare. In the same year, the Porritt Report suggested the NHS should break down the divisions between primary, secondary and community care, but the administrative structure was to remain intact until 1974.

The major reorganisation of that year – devised by a Conservative Government, but introduced by a Labour one – saw the formation in England of 14 regional health authorities and 90 area health authorities, which managed 206 district management teams. Teaching hospitals lost their separate status, while family practitioner committees were set up to oversee primary care. Community health councils were introduced to represent patients. Meanwhile, Scotland abolished its regional tier and set up central service organisations to carry out its functions. In the previous year, Northern Ireland had created the four health and social services boards that still survive but are due to be dissolved in 2008. The Welsh Hospital Board and 15 hospital management committees were replaced by eight health authorities coterminous with new local authorities. Everywhere, consensus management was the ruling philosophy.

England's area health authorities were short-lived, abolished in the next reorganisation of 1982 – devised and implemented by a Conservative Government – which created 192 district health authorities in their stead. Government dissatisfaction with consensus management – perceived to have given professional groups a veto over change – led to the beginning of a cultural upheaval with the Griffiths Report of 1983, which recommended general management replace consensus from top to bottom. In England and Wales, general managers at regional, district and unit level superseded consensus management teams, while an NHS Management Board within the Department of Health co-ordinated management nationally. Scotland and Northern Ireland followed suit a year later.

Funding crises and further reform

Repeated funding crises in the late 1980s – compounding underfunding from the 1970s – led to Prime Minister Margaret Thatcher's year-long review of the service that culminated in *Working for patients*, the 1989 white paper which heralded the introduction of the NHS internal market in 1991 in England, a year later in Scotland and Wales and subsequently in Northern Ireland. The 'purchasers' of healthcare – health authorities and some GP practices that became known as 'fundholders' – were separated from the 'providers' such as hospitals, ambulance and community services, which were formed into NHS trusts with a measure of self-government to compete with each other. The NHS Management Board became the NHS Executive, regional health authorities were reduced in number and family practitioner committees were replaced with family health services authorities.

In 1996, England's regional health authorities were swept away altogether in favour of regional offices of the NHS Executive, run by civil servants rather than NHS staff. Unified health authorities were created from the old districts and family health services authorities. In Wales, the nine existing health authorities and 18 family practitioner authorities were reconfigured into five new health authorities.

Into the 21st century

Pledging to abolish the internal market and GP fundholding on its election in 1997, the Labour Government sought a 'third way' of running the NHS, based on partnership and performance management. It involved yet more reorganisation. In England 500 primary care groups (later to become 300 primary care trusts, with additional powers) subsumed fundholding, and new bodies such as the National Institute for Clinical Excellence and Commission for Health Improvement (succeeded by the Healthcare Commission) took prominent roles. Health action zones were to encourage co-operation between health and social services, while community health services trusts were generally merged with PCGs. Wales established local health groups to replace fundholding, while Scotland introduced local healthcare co-operatives and its own version of primary care trusts. Devolution in 1999 meant the NHS in Scotland, Wales and Northern Ireland began to diverge – quite markedly in some policy areas – from the service in England.

The persistence of funding crises led to a large NHS spending increase in the 2000 Budget and further reform outlined in the NHS Plan later that year. The Wanless review's costing of future health needs led to another massive increase in the 2002 Budget and further waves of reform. Yet more restructuring came with the advent of 28 strategic health authorities in England, replacing the 100 unified health authorities; the SHAs were reduced to ten and the 300 PCTs halved in number in 2006. Other initiatives – such as patient choice, payment by results and foundation trusts – are still working their way through the system. Restructuring took place in Wales in 2004, in Scotland in 2005 and is being phased in up to 2008 in Northern Ireland.

Milestones

1946   NHS Act becomes law
1948   NHS begins
         First successful internal heart surgery
         Introduction of streptomycin for TB
1952   First prescription charge introduced
1953   Heart-lung machine invented
1954   First kidney transplant
1958   Smoking identified as cause of lung cancer
1959   Polio immunisation introduced
         Mental Health Act signals reform of long-stay institutions
1961   Contraceptive pill available on the NHS
1962   The Hospital Plan published
         Porritt recommends unification of hospitals, health authorities and general practices
1967   Abortion Act becomes law
1968   Britain's first successful heart transplant
1973   First CAT scan
1974   Regional and area health authorities, family practitioner committees and community health councils established
1979   Royal Commission on the NHS publishes its report
1980   Black reports on health inequalities
1982   Area health authorities abolished and 192 district health authorities created
1983   Griffiths recommends introduction of general management
         Private contractors tender for NHS cleaning, catering and laundering services

1984	AIDS virus discovered
	'Limited list' of drugs introduced to encourage generic prescribing
1985	Cervical screening programme begins
1986	National campaign to prevent the spread of AIDS
1988	Department of Health and Social Security split into two separate departments
1989	*Working for patients* white paper heralds the internal market
1991	Patient's Charter introduced
1993	Trade union Unison created from merger of NUPE, NALGO and COHSE
1994	14 regional health authorities reduced to eight
1997	NHS Primary Care Act
1999	Scottish Parliament, Welsh Assembly and NI Assembly take responsibility for NHS
2000	NHS Plan published
	Our national health published in Scotland
	GP Harold Shipman convicted of murdering 15 patients
2002	Wanless Report on future healthcare spending needs
2003	Community health councils abolished in England
	NHS Wales restructured
2004	First foundation trusts established
	NHS Improvement Plan published
	Choosing health public health white paper published
	NHSScotland abolishes trusts
2005	*Creating a patient-led* NHS published
	NHSScotland creates community health partnerships
	Reorganisation of health and social care in Northern Ireland announced
	Delivering for health white paper published in Scotland
2006	*Our health, our care, our say* white paper published in England
	28 strategic health authorities reduced to ten and 303 PCTs reduced to 152
	Scotland bans smoking in public places
2007	England, Wales and Northern Ireland ban smoking in public places.

An A–Z of the NHS

advocacy where a person acts as a champion for a patient or carer. An advocate could be employed to do this or it could be one of a range of people including a pharmacist, doctor, voluntary worker or a carer.

Audit Scotland responsible for securing the audit of NHS bodies and carrying out value-for-money studies since 2000.

benchmarking a process whereby organisations identify best performers in order to improve their own performance.

best value performance indicators measures of performance set by central Government departments since the duty of best value on local authorities came into effect in 1999, requiring authorities to continuously improve the efficiency, effectiveness and economy of their service delivery.

better services for vulnerable people requires agencies to work together to produce joint investment plans for older people, adults with mental health problems, people with learning disabilities and for welfare to work for disabled people.

British Medical Association professional association of doctors, acting as a trade union, scientific and educational body and publisher. Some 80 per cent of Britain's doctors are members.
www.bma.org.uk

Building capacity and partnership in care 2001 agreement between the statutory and independent social care sector, healthcare and housing sectors about placing older people in care homes or giving them other forms of support. Government investment of £300 million during 2001–03 aimed to reduce admissions and treatment and stabilise the home care sector with longer-term commissioning.

Caldicott guardian all NHS organisations must appoint a Caldicott guardian to safeguard the confidentiality of patient information, as do all councils with a social services responsibility. They must be:
- a member of the organisation's management board
- a senior health professional
- responsible for promoting clinical governance in the organisation.

The Caldicott principles apply in addition to the requirements of the Data Protection Act 1998.

Calman-Hine Report set out in 1995 a tiered network of care for cancer patients to ensure that care is of a uniformly high standard.

Campbell Collaboration international organisation that seeks to provide evidence of what works in public policy and of how, why and under what conditions policies work or fail.
www.campbellcollaboration.org

capital charges internal NHS charges (depreciation and interest) made against land, buildings and fixed assets.

Care Direct project since 2002, a DH and local council service for people over 60, their carers and relatives. It aims to make it easier for people to get information and help concerning social care, health, housing and social security benefits when they need it. There is a free phone (0800 444 000), local help-desks in pilot areas and a website.
www.caredirect.gov.uk

Care Programme Approach (CPA) ensures that PCTs and social services departments have systematic arrangements for assessing the health and social care needs of mentally ill people, and that people referred to secondary services get appropriate care, including an individual treatment plan.

Carers (Recognition and Services) Act 1995 gives people who provide substantial care on a regular basis the right to ask for an assessment from social services.

Caring about Carers 1999 national strategy supporting an estimated 6 million carers. Its main features are:
- grants to allow English local authorities to help carers take a break
- credits towards a second pension
- council tax reductions for more disabled people and their carers
- more carer-friendly employment policies
- support for young carers, including those at school.

case mix the mixture of clinical conditions and severity of condition met in patients in a particular healthcare setting.

clinical audit a cyclical measurement and evaluation by health professionals of the clinical standards they are achieving.

clinical directorate a unit within an NHS trust providing specific clinical services, frequently led by a consultant.

Cochrane collaboration an international network, of which the UK Cochrane Centre is a member, that builds, maintains and disseminates up-to-date information from the systematic review of healthcare trials.

Commission for Social Care Inspection (CSCI) carries out work previously undertaken by the Social Services Inspectorate, the SSI/Audit Commission joint review team and the social care functions of the National Care Standards Commission.

Data Protection Act 1998 governs processing of personal data about all living people in the UK. It sets out principles for handling information that all data controllers must comply with. Its remit includes access to health records of living people and patients' rights to have inaccurate information corrected.

emergency planning plan outlining how to deal with a serious incident, such as a major road accident, rail crash, bomb incident or chemical spill. Each level and part of the NHS has an emergency plan, which must relate to the emergency plans of other agencies, such as local authorities, police and fire services.

enforcement protocol (smoking) developed in conjunction with local authorities to reduce under-age tobacco sales. Local authorities have to take enforcement action at least once each year.

European Medicines Evaluation Agency authorises the use of medicinal products in the European Union and works with national medicines regulatory bodies (see also Medicines and Healthcare Products Regulatory Agency).

extended schools schools with a wider role to provide family, social care and health services.

Fair shares for all review of resource allocation for NHSScotland chaired by Sir John Arbuthnott that led to a new formula being adopted.

finished consultant episode completion of a patient's period of care under a consultant, after which they are either discharged or transferred to another consultant.

Food Standards Agency charged with protecting health in relation to food, with powers to act throughout the food chain to develop policies. Advises consumers, ministers and the food industry on all aspects of food safety and standards. FSA also operates in Scotland and Wales.

Funding learning and development for the healthcare workforce 2002 DH paper recommending a single integrated budget designed to support learning by health professionals across the board.

General Social Care Council promotes high standards of conduct, practice and training for social workers. The Council, which began in 2001, has established a code of practice and a register of social care workers.

Health action zones (HAZs) partnerships between the NHS, local authorities, the voluntary and private sectors and local communities. Launched by the DH in 1998, the HAZ initiative was concerned with new ways of tackling health inequalities in some of the most deprived areas.

Health and Safety Commission responsible for administering the Health and Safety at Work Act 1974. Its role is to ensure risks from work activities are properly controlled. It reviews health and safety legislation and makes proposals for changes.

Health and Safety Executive assists the Health and Safety Commission in its functions. It has specific statutory responsibilities, including enforcement of health and safety law. Its staff includes inspectors, policy advisers, lawyers, technologists and scientific and medical experts.

health and social care awards annual award scheme for NHS and social services staff, which recognises outstanding achievement.

health service circular (HSC) formal method of communication between the DH and the rest of the NHS.

healthy schools initiative launched in 1998, aims to raise the awareness of children, teachers, governors, parents and the wider community to the opportunities that exist in schools for improving health. A website and healthy schools network support the initiative.

hospital consultants take full responsibility for the clinical care of patients. Most head a team, or 'firm', of doctors in training. The team may include specialist registrars as well as clinical assistants, hospital practitioners, associate specialists and staff-grade doctors.

hotel costs the accommodation costs of keeping a patient in hospital, excluding treatment costs.

Human Fertilisation and Embryology Authority since 1991, licenses and monitors NHS and private fertility clinics. It is charged with ensuring research is carried out responsibly. HFEA is to be merged into the new Regulatory Authority for Fertility and Tissue by 2008.

Human Genetics Commission since 1999, advises on the social, ethical and legal implications of developments in genetics and their likely impact on health and healthcare. It engages the public in considering these questions.

Human Rights Act 1998 incorporates into domestic law the European Convention on Human Rights. The intention is to embed values of fairness, respect for human dignity and inclusiveness in the heart of public services. The law prohibits any public authority acting in a way that is incompatible with a Convention right. Since its introduction the NHS has seen a number of cases dealing with the right to life and the right to die with dignity, as well as challenges to the way mentally ill people are treated.

independent mental capacity advocate (IMCA) introduced by the Mental Capacity Act 2005 to support and represent the most vulnerable people who are not always able to make their own decisions about their welfare, finances or healthcare.

Information and Statistics Division leading source of health data in Scotland.

Joint Futures Agenda a collaboration set up in 1999 between NHSScotland and local government in areas such as community care, health improvement and social inclusion.

learning disability incomplete intellectual development, sometimes accompanied by social or emotional problems. The 2001 white paper *Valuing people: a new strategy for learning disability for the 21st century* aims to help people with learning disabilities to live as independently as possible.

magnetic resonance imaging (MRI) sophisticated and expensive equipment that uses magnetic fields to create images of the body to aid diagnosis.

Managing for excellence in the NHS 2002 paper by the then NHS chief executive calling for NHS management to be strengthened by:
- implementing the code of conduct for NHS managers
- supporting managers and leaders
- investment in development
- bringing on talent to create more skilled, experienced and diverse leadership
- developing senior management and succession planning
- reducing top-down burdens and encouraging diversity.

market forces supplement means of topping up the pay of selected staff in areas of labour market shortages.

Medicines and Healthcare Products Regulatory Agency formed in 2003 from the merger of the Medicines Control Agency and the Medical Devices Agency. It is responsible for regulating medicines and healthcare products. Its main objective is to protect public health by ensuring medicines, healthcare products and medical equipment are safe (see also European Medicines Evaluation Agency.

medicines management the delivery of medicines to patients based on their needs. Aims to enable patients to get maximum benefit from medicines while reducing waste, and involves pharmacists working more closely with other health professionals.

MEDLINE an electronic database providing abstracts of thousands of biomedical studies.
www.nlm.nih.gov

Mental Capacity Act 2005 governs decision-making on behalf of adults who have lost mental capacity or where the incapacitating condition has been present since birth.

Mental Health Act 1983 governs the admission of people to psychiatric hospital against their will, their rights while detained, discharge from hospital and aftercare. The Act applies in England and Wales. Divided into sections, the term 'being sectioned' means to be compulsorily admitted to hospital.

Mental Health Act code of practice good-practice guidance for professionals and managers implementing the Mental Health Act.

Mental Health Act Commission special health authority responsible for protecting the interests of patients detained in England and Wales. To be abolished in 2007.

Mental Health Act managers NHS trust non-executive directors who have power under the 1983 Mental Health Act to admit or discharge mentally ill patients.

mental health review tribunal hears appeals against detention under the Mental Health Act. It consists of two distinct bodies: the judicial tribunal responsible for hearing applications concerning people detained under the Act, and the secretariat, which administers the tribunals. Tribunals consist of medical, legal and lay members.

national beds inquiry confirmed that the NHS needed more hospital beds in the right places to work quickly and efficiently. In 2000/01 there were 135,794 general and acute NHS hospital beds in England. The NHS Plan stipulated an increase of 7,000 by 2004, with 2,100 in acute wards.

National Horizon Scanning Centre run by Birmingham University, this provides advance notice of significant new and emerging technologies to the DH.
www.pcpoh.bham.ac.uk

National Institute for Mental Health in England part of the Care Services Improvement Partnership sponsored by the Department of Health, it helps local development centres and national programmes implement policy and resolve local challenges in developing mental health services. Launched in 2002, NIMHE takes a lead in connecting mental health research, development, delivery, monitoring and review.

National Primary Care Research and Development Centre a multidisciplinary centre in Manchester set up in 1995 to improve NHS primary and community healthcare by applying knowledge relevant to the funding, organisation and delivery of health services.
www.npcrdc.man.ac.uk

National Treatment Agency (for Substance Misuse) launched in 2001 to provide services to drug misusers through pooled budgets from health and other agencies. It is encouraging good practice, setting standards and monitoring performance.

neighbourhood renewal *A new commitment to neighbourhood renewal* (2001), a national strategy action plan, sets out a joined-up approach to tackling the social and economic problems in the most rundown neighbourhoods – including low educational achievement, crime, unemployment and poor housing.

NHS Blood and Transplant since October 2005 a special health authority that promotes the donation of blood and organs, co-ordinates a 24-hour organ-matching and allocation service and arranges and keeps track of the collection, preparation and distribution of blood. It replaced the National Blood Authority and UK Transplant.
www.nhssbt.nhs.uk

NHS Cancer Plan 2000 provides the fullest statement of the Government's comprehensive national programme for investment and reform of cancer services in England.

NHS Clinical Governance Support Team currently under review, it helps organisations implement clinical governance with information, advice and development programmes.
www.cgsupport.nhs.uk

NHS Plus NHS network that provides – for a fee – occupational health services to public and private sector employers.
www.nhsplus.nhs.uk

nicotine replacement therapy doubles the chances of smokers quitting successfully. Available on NHS prescription from 2001.

Nolan principles seven principles governing public life drawn up by Lord Nolan's committee in 1995: selflessness, integrity, objectivity, accountability, openness, honesty and leadership. They are used to guide the appointment of non-executive directors.

palliative care the active total care of patients whose disease no longer responds to curative treatment. Should neither hasten nor postpone death. It pays equal attention to the physical, psychological, social and spiritual aspects of care of patients and those close to them.

paramedic ambulance personnel qualified to provide pre-hospital procedures and care.

pathology a consultant advisory service supported by laboratory facilities where specimens of blood, urine, tissue etc, taken from patients are analysed.

patient environment action teams DH teams which since 2000 have audited progress in implementing a nationwide clean-up campaign to improve the cleanliness and environment for NHS hospital patients.

patient pathway the route followed by the patient into, through and out of NHS and social care services. It can involve referral from primary care to hospital, visits to hospital departments and specialties, a pathway through a clinical network, or the experience of joint NHS and social care in the community.

patients' prospectus document to be published by every primary care trust as part of the NHS Plan outlining the views they have received from patients in the previous year and the action taken as a result.

pay-bed a bed in an NHS hospital occupied by a patient who pays the whole cost of accommodation, medical and other services.

pay review body independent panels which recommend pay awards for NHS staff such as doctors and dentists, nurses and allied health professionals. Appointments to the pay review body are the responsibility of the Prime Minister. Their recommendations are submitted to the Secretary of State for Health who can authorise the proposed pay rises.

pharmaceutical industry competitiveness taskforce set up by the Prime Minister to see what action needed to be taken to ensure the UK remained an attractive place for the industry to locate. Reported in 2001 and referred to the need to involve the industry in the development of NHS services.

Positively Diverse a national benchmarking programme to develop the NHS workforce across local communities. It brings together NHS organisations, local government and higher education, and is looking at how to support the capacity and skills needed to respond to and deal with diversity.

primary care investment plan each PCT must prepare a plan covering a three-year investment cycle. The PCIP is designed to protect spending in general medical services and primary care and to assist planning for further improvement of primary care services. It must be consistent with the local delivery plan.

Pursuing Perfection (P2) an international programme to improve outcomes for patients across whole systems. The programme is led by the Institute for Healthcare Improvement in Boston, USA, and involves more than 13 healthcare systems around the world.

quality-adjusted life year a measure which assesses variations in the quality of life for the patient resulting from an intervention, in relation to cost and length of life. Used for measuring the clinical and cost-effectiveness of interventions.

quality and outcomes framework a system of standards, incentives and assessment for GP practices.

Regulatory Authority for Fertility and Tissue (RAFT) from 2008 will regulate assisted reproduction, embryo research and the use of human tissue, replacing the Human Fertilisation and Embryology Authority and the Human Tissue Authority.

Royal College of Nursing the world's largest professional union of nurses. The RCN is run by nurses, it campaigns on behalf of the profession and helps to develop nursing practice and standards of care. Through the RCN Institute it provides higher education and promotes research, quality and practice development.
www.rcn.org.uk

Royal Commission on long-term care body that looked into the funding of long-term care for older people (*With respect to old age*, 1999).

Saving lives: our healthier nation public health white paper, published in July 1999, set objectives to improve the health of the population as a whole and especially the worst-off in society. It set up public health observatories and dealt with issues such as teenage pregnancies, sexual health, food safety and water fluoridation.

Scottish Audit of Surgical Mortality audit unique in the UK, covering all surgical specialties and almost all consultant surgeons and anaesthetists. SASM identifies all deaths that occur under the care of a surgeon, whether or not there has been an operation.
www.sasm.org.uk

single regeneration budget funding available to areas of severe need, revamped to give greater support to community development.

smoking control network an umbrella organisation comprising health charities, the medical profession, pharmaceutical companies and Government, which campaigns to reduce smoking-related deaths.

standardised mortality ratio the number of deaths in a given year as a percentage of those expected.

starter homes initiative funding to help the NHS ease staffing shortages in parts of London and the south.

systematic review a review of clinical literature in a particular field that has set explicit tests for whether research is valuable enough to be included in an overview of the area.

telemedicine the use of communications systems (such as electronic networks and VDUs) to provide remote diagnosis, advice, treatment and monitoring. Being used in both primary and hospital settings.

Transfer of Undertakings (Protection of Employment) Regulations 1981 regulations designed to ensure that employees transferred from one employer to another maintain employment rights.

Unfinished business 2002 report by the chief medical officer on modernising the senior house officer grade. Calls for more structured training.

UNISON public services and essential industries trade union. It represents employees in local government, healthcare, the voluntary sector and elsewhere. The largest trade union in the NHS.

Valuing people 2001 white paper on learning disabilities, based on people having their rights as citizens respected, inclusion in local communities, choice in daily life and real chances to be independent.

whole-system planning strategic planning and commissioning across a range of services and organisational boundaries. Deals with the impact that changes in one part of the system, whether health and social care or housing, are likely to have on other parts.

World Health Organisation international non-governmental body, primarily concerned with promoting co-operation in strengthening health and healthcare worldwide.
www.who.int

Acronym buster

ABPI	Association of the British Pharmaceutical Industry
AC	Audit Commission
ACAD	ambulatory care and diagnostic unit
ACDA	Advisory Committee on Distinction Awards (consultants)
ACDP	Advisory Committee on Dangerous Pathogens
ACEVO	Association of Chief Executives of Voluntary Organisations
ACGT	Advisory Committee on Generic Testing
ACRA	Advisory Committee on Resource Allocation
ADSS	Association of Directors of Social Services
A&E	accident and emergency
AHP	allied health profession(al)
AM	Assembly Member (Wales)
ASCT	Asylum Seeker Co-ordination Team
BAMM	British Association of Medical Managers
BMA	British Medical Association
BSC	Business Services Centre (NHS Wales)
CAMHS	child and adolescent mental health services
CAT	computerised axial tomography (scan)
CCIT	consultant contract implementation team
CDO	chief dental officer
CEAC	Clinical and Excellence Awards Committee (Northern Ireland)
CEMACH	Confidential Enquiry into Maternal and Child Health
CGST	(NHS) clinical governance support team
CHAI	Commission for Healthcare Audit and Inspection (previous name for the Healthcare Commission)
CHC	community health council
CHCP	community health and care partnership (Scotland)
CHD	coronary heart disease
CHIQ	Centre for Health Information Quality
CHMS	central health and miscellaneous services
CHP	community health partnership (Scotland)
CIMP	clinical information management programme
CIO	chief information officer
CIP	cost improvement programme
CME	continuing medical education
CMHT	community mental health team

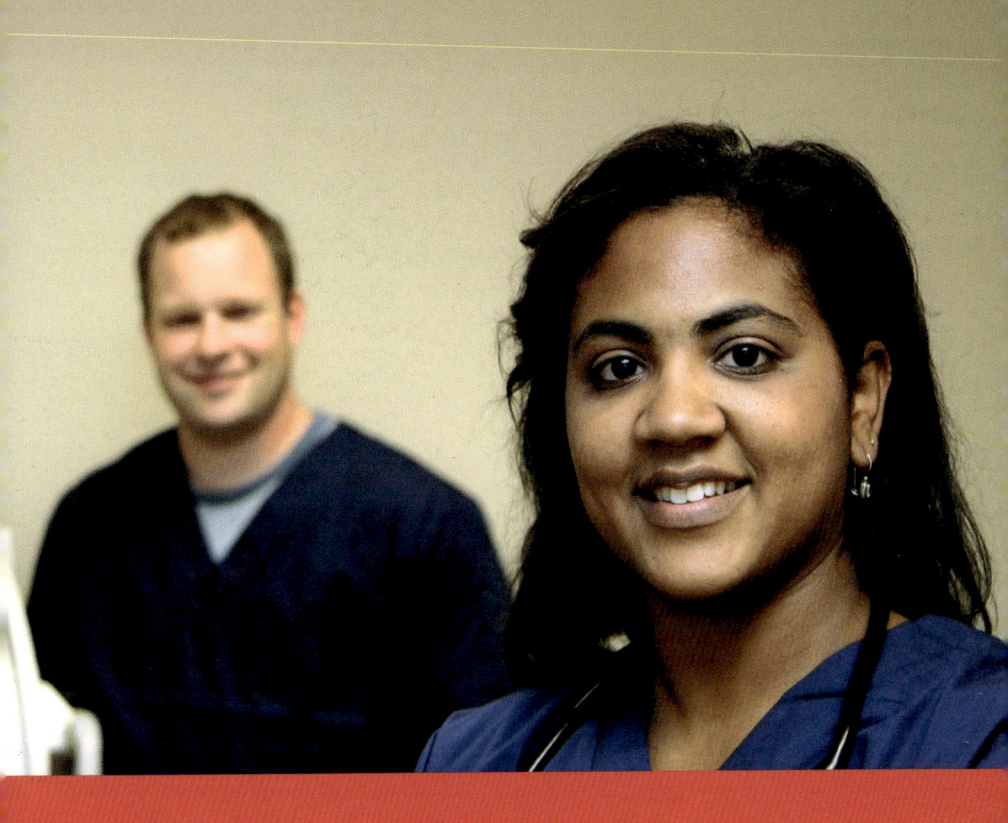

HEALTHY PARTNERSHIPS »

Atos Healthcare is dedicated to creating healthy partnerships with the NHS to improve patient care and the wellbeing of society. Our primary care, occupational health and diagnostic services combine the highest standards of clinical excellence, innovation and value for money.

Atos Healthcare works as a partner for change with the NHS at a local, regional and national level, through the unique combination of business consulting, IT and healthcare services.

For further information please call 020 7830 4931

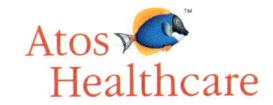

Atos Healthcare

CMO	chief medical officer
CNO	chief nursing officer
CNST	Clinical Negligence Scheme for Trusts
COMARE	Committee on Medical Aspects of Radiation in the Environment
COMEAP	Committee on the Medical Effects of Air Pollutants
COSLA	Convention of Scottish Local Authorities
CPA	care programme approach
CPD	continuing professional development
CPPIH	Commission for Patient and Public Involvement in Health
CPR	Child Protection Register
CRD	(NHS) Centre for Research and Dissemination
CRHP	Council for the Regulation of Healthcare Professionals
CRS	Care Records Service
CSA	Common Services Agency
CSM	Committee on the Safety of Medicines
CSR	comprehensive spending review
CTO	compulsory treatment order
DAT	drug action team
DCLG	Department for Communities and Local Government
DDRB	doctors' and dentists' (pay) review body
DEFRA	Department for Environment, Food and Rural Affairs
DfES	Department for Education and Skills
DFT	distance from target
DGH	district general hospital
DH or DoH	Department of Health
DHSSPS	Department of Health, Social Services and Public Safety (Northern Ireland)
DPB	Dental Practice Board
DPH	director of public health
DPR	Data Protection Registrar
DSU	day surgery unit
DTC	diagnosis and treatment centre
EBH	evidence-based healthcare
EBM	evidence-based medicine
EBS	emergency bed service
ECHR	European Convention on Human Rights
ECR	extra-contractual referral
EFL	external financing limit

e-GIF	(electronic) Government Interoperability Framework
EHR	electronic health record
ENT	ear, nose and throat
EO	employers' organisation
EPR	electronic patient record
EPS	electronic prescription service
ERDIP	electronic record development and implementation programme
ESR	electronic staff record
ETP	electronic transmission of prescriptions
EWTD	European working-time directive
FCE	finished consultant episode
FHS	family health services
FMP	financial management programme
FOI	freedom of information
FSA	Food Standards Agency
GDC	General Dental Council
GMC	General Medical Council
GMS	general medical services
GPSI or GPWSI	general practitioner with a special interest
GSCC	General Social Care Council
GTAC	Gene Therapy Advisory Committee
GUM	genito-urinary medicine (clinic)
GWC	General Whitley Council
HA	health authority
HAZ	health action zone
HB	health board
HBG	health benefit group
HCC	Healthcare Commission
HCHS	hospital and community health services
HDA	Health Development Agency
HDL	Health Department letter
HEFCE	Higher Education Funding Council for England
HES	hospital episode statistics
HFEA	Human Fertilisation and Embryology Authority
HIA	health impact assessment
HIMP	health improvement and modernisation plan
HIW	Health Inspectorate Wales

HLC	healthy living centre
HMO	health maintenance organisation (US)
HOWIS	Health of Wales Information Service
HPA	Health Protection Agency
HPC	Health Professions Council
HPMA	Healthcare People Management Association
HPSS	Health and Personal Social Services (Northern Ireland)
HRG	healthcare resource group
HSC	health service circular; (House of Commons) Health Select Committee
HSCA	Health and Social Care Authority (Northern Ireland)
HSCI	health service cost index
HSCT	Health and Social Care Trust (Northern Ireland)
HSSB	Health and Social Services Board (Northern Ireland)
HSSC	Health and Social Services Council (Northern Ireland)
HTA	health technology assessment
IC	information commissioner
ICAS	Independent Complaints Advocacy Service
ICD	international classification of diseases
ICP	integrated care pathway
ICRS	integrated care records service
ICT	information and communication technology
ICU	intensive care unit
ILA	individual learning account
IMCA	independent mental capacity advocate
IM&T	information management and technology
IP	inpatient
IPR	individual performance review
IPU	(Department of Health) Information Policy Unit
IRP	independent reconfiguration panel
ISB	(NHS) Information Standards Board
ISD	Information and Statistics Division (Scotland)
IWL	Improving Working Lives
JIPs	joint investment plans
LAA	local area agreement
LAL	local authority letter
LASSL	local authority social services letter
LDP	local delivery plan
LGA	Local Government Association

LHB	local health board
LHC	local health council
LHCC	local healthcare co-operative
LHG	local health group
LHP	local health plan
LHSCG	Local Health and Social Care Group (Northern Ireland)
LIS	local implementation strategy
LPSA	local public service agreement
LSP	local strategic partnership; local service provider
LTA	long-term agreement
MCN	managed clinical network
MCO	managed care organisation
MFS	market forces supplement
MHAC	Mental Health Act Commission
MHRA	Medicines and Healthcare Products Regulatory Agency
MHRT	mental health review tribunal
MLA	Member of the Legislative Assembly (Northern Ireland)
MMC	Modernising Medical Careers
MMR	measles, mumps, rubella
MRC	Medical Research Council
MRI	magnetic resonance imaging
MRSA	methicillin-resistant *Staphylococcus aureus*
MSP	Member of the Scottish Parliament
N3	new national network (broadband)
NAO	National Audit Office
NASP	national application service provider
NatPaCT	National primary and care trust (development programme)
NAW	National Assembly for Wales
NBA	National Blood Authority
NBAP	national booked admissions programme
NBI	national beds inquiry
NCAA	National Clinical Assessment Authority
NCASP	National Clinical Audit Support Programme
NCE	national confidential enquiry
NCEPOD	National Confidential Enquiry into Perioperative Deaths
NCSC	National Care Standards Commission
NCVO	National Council for Voluntary Organisations
NDPB	non-departmental public body

NED	non-executive director
NeLH	National electronic Library for Health
NES	NHS Education for Scotland
nGMS	new general medical services (contract)
NHSI	NHS Institute for Innovation and Improvement
NHSL	NHS Logistics
NHSLA	NHS Litigation Authority
NHS LIFT	NHS Local Improvement Finance Trust
NHS QIS	NHS Quality Improvement Scotland
NHST	NHS trust
NIA	Northern Ireland Assembly
NIC	national insurance contribution
NICE	National Institute for Health and Clinical Excellence
NIMHE	National Institute for Mental Health in England
NLIAH	National Leadership and Innovation Agency for Healthcare (Wales)
NMC	Nursing and Midwifery Council
NOF	National Opportunities Fund
NPfIT	National Programme for IT (in the NHS)
NPG	national priorities guidance
NPHS	National Public Health Service (Wales)
NPSA	National Patient Safety Agency
NRAC	NHSScotland Resource Allocation Committee
NRCI	national reference cost index
NRPB	National Radiological Protection Board
NRT	nicotine replacement therapy
NSCAG	national specialist commissioning advisory group
NSF	national service framework
NSRC	national schedule of reference costs
NSS	National Services Scotland
NTA	National Treatment Agency (for Substance Misuse)
NTO	national training organisation
OAT	out-of-area treatment
OCMO	Office of the Chief Medical Officer (Wales)
ODP	operating department practitioner
OHE	Office of Health Economics
ONS	Office for National Statistics
OP	outpatient
OSC	(local authority) overview and scrutiny committee

OT	occupational therapist/therapy
OTC	over-the-counter
PAC	public accounts committee
PACS	picture archiving and communications system
PAF	performance assessment framework
PALS	patient advice and liaison service
PbR	payment by results
PCG	primary care group
PCIP	primary care investment plan
PCO	primary care organisation
PCT	primary care trust
PDP	personal development plan
PEC	professional executive committee (of PCT)
PFI	private finance initiative
PHeL	Public Health electronic Library
PHO	public health observatory
PMETB	Postgraduate Medical Education and Training Board
PMS	personal medical services
PPA	Prescription Pricing Authority
PPF	priorities and planning framework
PPI	patient and public involvement
PPO	preferred provider organisation
PPP	public–private partnership
PPRS	Pharmaceutical Price Regulation Scheme
PRB	pay review body
PSA	public service agreement
QA	quality assurance
QALY	quality-adjusted life year
QMAS	quality management and analysis system
RAWP	resource allocation working party
RCN	Royal College of Nursing
RCP	Royal College of Physicians
RCPE	Royal College of Physicians of Edinburgh
RCPSG	Royal College of Physicians and Surgeons of Glasgow
RCS	Royal College of Surgeons
RCSE	Royal College of Surgeons of Edinburgh
RCT	randomised controlled trial
RTA	road traffic accident

SACDA	Scottish Advisory Committee on Distinction Awards
SARS	severe acute respiratory syndrome
SAS	Scottish Ambulance Service
SASM	Scottish Audit of Surgical Mortality
SCVO	Scottish Council for Voluntary Organisations
SEHD	Scottish Executive Health Department
SEU	Social Exclusion Unit
SFA	statement of fees and allowances
SHA	strategic health authority; special health authority
SHARE	Scottish health authorities revenue equalisation
SHO	senior house officer
SHOW	Scottish Health on the Web
SHRINE	Strategic Human Resources Information Network
SIGN	Scottish Intercollegiate Guidelines Network
SLA	service level agreement
SMAC	Standing Medical Advisory Committee
SMR	standardised mortality ratio
SNMAC	Standing Nursing and Midwifery Advisory Committee
SNOMED	systematised nomenclature of medicine
SRB	single regeneration budget
SSA	standard spending assessment
SSC	shared service centre
SSI	Social Services Inspectorate
TEL	trust executive letter
TUPE	Transfer of Undertakings (Protection of Employment) Regulations
VFM	value for money
WCH	Wales Centre for Health
WDC	workforce development confederation
WHO	World Health Organisation
WIsH	Welsh Innovations in Healthcare
WTD	working-time directive

This list can be found in electronic form on the NHS Confederation website at www.nhsconfed.org/pocketguide

# Index

This index relates primarily to Part 1 of the pocket guide and does not extensively cover topics included in the A–Z section commencing on page 210. Therefore, when looking up a topic, there may be occasions when users might refer to the A–Z as well as this index.

alternative provider medical services (APMS) 20
ambulance services 56, 58
ambulance trusts 57
'annual health check' 83, 86
annual performance rating 85
Appointments Commission 38
arm's-length bodies 16
asylum seekers 104, 159, 160

beds 51, 55
Big Lottery Fund 104
bullying 132

capital funding 109
capital investment 109
care-closer-to-home pilot sites 40
Care Services Improvement Partnership (CSIP) 27
care services, Scotland 172
care trusts 25
carers 62
Centre for Public Scrutiny 147
charges, NHS 102
chief medical officer 16
children's commissioner 145
children's issues 12
children's services 27, 145, 153
children's services director 26
children's trust 26
Choose and Book 137

clinical governance 80
clinical negligence procedures 86–8
clinical networks 26
Clostridium difficile 76
code of conduct for NHS managers 94
code of practice for promoting NHS services 31
Commission for Social Care Inspection 82
commissioning 20
 lead 145
 practice-based 22
community health councils 66, 67, 183
community health partnerships 18, 143, 167
community health services 48
community hospitals 40, 50, 143
community matrons 48, 127
community nurses 48
community pharmacies 46
Compact, the 149
complaints manager 97
complaints procedure 40, 96
 independent review 97
 number of complaints 98
comprehensive spending review 104
consultant episodes 118
consultants' contract 130
continuing professional development 93
contracting 19
core standards 83, 84

231

Council for Healthcare Regulatory Excellence 91, 92
cross-border healthcare 33
CRS Registration Authority 137

delayed discharge 148
dental services 45, 88
 charges 103
Department of Health (DH)
 chief professional officers 15
 health committee 11
 management structure 14
 permanent secretary 13, 15
developmental standards 83
DH board 15
director for equality and human rights 159
drugs bill 118

efficiency savings 116
eHealth IM&T strategy 177
electronic care record 69
electronic prescription service 138
emergency care practitioner 58
equality and diversity 132
European Union 33
Expert Patient, The 67

foundation trusts 23, 24, 97, 109
 boards 37
Freedom of Information Act 98
Future Healthcare Network 49

General Medical Council 91, 124
general medical services (GMS)
 contract 19, 59, 129–30
governance
 corporate 81

financial 81
 information 81
 research 81
GP patient survey 95
GP practices 19, 22, 39, 88, 95, 106, 111, 130
 staff 39
GP services 20
GPs 19, 22, 28, 39, 128, 130
 special interest 41

Health Development Agency 87
Health Professions Council 90
Health Protection Agency 156
Health Service Commissioner 12
health service cost index (HSCI) 117
health trainers 153, 159
health visitors 48
Healthcare Commission 74, 76, 83, 85, 95, 97, 131
Healthy Living Centres 161

Independent Complaints Advocacy Services (ICAS) 98
independent hospitals 28
Independent Reconfiguration Panel 54
independent sector 28
infectious diseases 158
Information Centre for Health and Social Care 141
ëinformation prescriptions' 40
Integrated Care Network 147
intermediate care 50
involving patients 64–66

job reductions 122

local area agreements 146
local authorities 23, 143–8

Index

local authority overview and scrutiny
  committees 54, 66
local commissioning groups 18, 143
local delivery plans (LDPs) 74
local health boards 18, 182
Local Involvement Networks (LINks) 66
local partnership forums 177
local patient surveys 96
local strategic partnerships 149
long-term conditions 51

managed clinical networks 168
maternity services 27
medicines 69, 119, 169
Mental Capacity Act 2005 64
mental health 25, 59–62
Mental Health Act Commission 82
Mental Health Bill 63
mental health law, revision of 63
mental health, NSF 62
mental health services 59–62
mental health trusts 24, 59
mental healthcare and race equality 63
Modernising Medical Careers 126
Monitor 24

N3: New National Network 138
National Clinical Assessment Service 89
national clinical directors 16
national director for patients and
  the public 67
National Institute for Health and
  Clinical Excellence (NICE) 87
National Leadership and Innovation
  Agency for Healthcare 192
National Library for Health 140
National PALS Development Group 66
National Patient Safety Agency 88

national patient surveys 95
National Programme for IT (NPfIT) 133,
  134, 135, 136
national schedule of reference costs 106
national service frameworks 83
National standards, local action 83
negligence claims 89
new providers 27
NHS
  funding 13, 111
  priorities 8
  resources, disposition of 116
  spending 8, 105, 111–15, 117
  structure 8–10
  underlying values 8
NHS Bank 114
NHS boards
  chair 34
  chief executive 36
  committees 36
  duties and responsibilities 32
  non-executive directors 35
NHS Business Services Authority 120
NHS Care Records Service (CRS) 136
NHS Careers 124
NHS Centre for Involvement 65
NHS chief executive 13
  report 13
  weekly bulletin 13
NHS Connecting for Health 136
NHS Counter Fraud Service 120
NHS Direct 43
NHS Direct Interactive 44
NHS Direct Online 44
NHS Elect 56
NHS Employers 123, 127
NHS Health Direct 44
NHS Institute for Innovation and

233

Improvement 128
NHS Jobs 127
NHS Knowledge and Skills 129
NHS Litigation Authority 88, 89, 129
NHS Local Improvement Finance Trust (LIFT) 111
NHS Logistics 120
NHSmail 139
NHS Modernisation Agency 128
NHSnet 138
NHS Networks 27
NHS number 140
NHS Numbers For Babies (NN4B) 140
NHS Patient Survey Programme Advice Centre 96
NHS Purchasing and Supply Agency 120
NHS Quality Improvement Scotland 87
NHS Redress Act 88
NHS Shared Business Services 118
NHS Supply Chain 120
NHS trusts 23
   in Scotland 23
   spending 114
NHS.uk 139
NHSweb 139
non-department public bodies 16
Northern Ireland
   health and social services 25
   Patient and Client Council 67
Northern Ireland Assembly 8, 11, 104
Northern Ireland's Department of Health, Social Services and Public Safety 13
nurses 22, 39, 41, 42, 48, 124
Nursing and Midwifery Council 90

obesity 153
older people 12, 25, 148
Ombudsman 12, 98, 100

one-stop health centres 41, 111
operations, numbers of 53
optical service review 48
opticians 47
Our health, our care, our say 40
overseas clinical teams 31
overseas treatment 31
overseas visitors 104
overview and scrutiny committees 146

partnership arrangements 142
Partnerships for Health 111
patient advice and liaison services (PALS) 66
patient and public involvement forums 66
patient choice 68
patient safety 84
payment by results 108
performance assessment 83–86
   framework 83
personal medical services (PMS) contract 20
Pharmaceutical Price Regulation Scheme (PPRS) 118
pharmacies 28
postgraduate education 124, 125, 126
practice-based commissioning 106
prescription charges 103, 189
primary care trusts (PCTs) 18–22, 28
   boards 36
   commissioning services 28
   resource allocation 105–6
   spending 114
PRIMIS+ 141
priorities and planning framework 73
prison healthcare 151
private finance initiative (PFI) 109
private sector 28, 88, 100

Acknowledgements

The NHS Confederation is grateful to all those involved in the production of this expanded edition of the *Pocket Guide*. Particular thanks are due to:
- our sponsor, Atos Origin
- all those who have supported the guide through advertising (listed below)
- those organisations that have kindly allowed us to reproduce diagrams and other materials
- Caroline Ball and John Cox for their expert editing and proof-reading
- Grade Design, for designing and typesetting this year's guide and PWS Design for their work on the front cover.

We are also grateful to our members and other customers who have provided valuable feedback on previous editions of the *Pocket Guide*, to enable us to make year-on-year improvements.

List of advertisers

Supplies Team	Inside front cover
Care Services Improvement Partnership (CSIP)	Page 179
Atos Healthcare	Page 223
Capsticks	Back cover

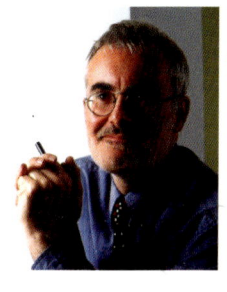

The author

Peter Davies is a freelance writer and editor. He has written extensively on health policy and management issues, for which he won a major award from the Medical Journalists Association. He was editor of *Health Service Journal* from 1993 to 2002, and has contributed a regular column to *Guardian Unlimited*. He is married with two children and lives in London.

Index

professional executive committee (PEC) 36
professional self-regulation 90–2
public accountability 34
public accounts committee 12
public administration committee 12
public health 151
  ill health prevention 155
  Wanless Report 155
  white paper 152
  workforce 154
public health observatories 161
public service agreement 71

Quality and Outcomes Framework 130

reconfiguring services, review of 53
Reforming Emergency Care 56
refugees 159
resource accounting and budgeting (RAB) 107
resources 13
  allocation 104–7
  disposition of 116
road accidents, recovering costs 103
  Compensation Recovery Unit 103
Royal Colleges 125

Scottish Executive Health Department 13, 164
Scottish Health Council 67
Scottish Parliament 8, 11, 104
Select Committees 11
service level agreement 23
sexual health services 153
Shipman Inquiry 91
sight test charges 103
smoking 153, 154, 159
social enterprises 30

DH social enterprise unit 30
  social enterprise fund 30
special health authorities 16
specialist nurses 48
staff
  morale 131
  numbers 121–2
Staff Governance Standard 176
strategic health authorities 17, 23, 121
stress 132
supersurgeries 41

teaching PCTs 22
third sector organisations 30
training 106, 121, 124–6
treatment centres 29, 54, 55, 56

UK Information Management & Technology Forum 136
undergraduate education 124

value for money 112
voluntary sector 23, 28

waiting times 75, 76, 108, 127
walk-in centres 42
Wanless Report 113
  report on public health 155
weighted capitation formula 106
Welsh Assembly 8, 11, 104
Welsh Health and Social Care Department 13
Whole Health Community Diagnostic Project 25
workforce planning 121
Workforce Review Team 121, 124
working people's health 152

Xansa 118

235